EMQs for
Medical Students
Volume 2
Second Edition

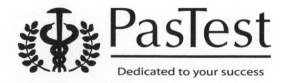

PasTest

Dedicated to your success

EMQs for
Medical Students
Volume 2
Second Edition

Adam Feather FRCP

Charles H Knowles BChir PhD FRCS (Gen Surg)

Jonathan Round BA MBBS MRCP

Paulo Domizio BSc MBBS FRCPath

Benjamin C T Field MBBS BMedSci MSc MRCP

John S P Lumley MS FRCS

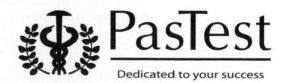

PasTest
Dedicated to your success

Egerton Court
Parkgate Estate
Knutsford
Cheshire
WA16 8DX

Telephone: 01565 752000

First Edition 2001
Reprinted 2002, 2003, 2007
Second Edition 2008
Reprinted 2008, 2009

ISBN: 1 905635 38 9
978 1905635 382

A catalogue record for this book is available from the British Library.

The information contained within this book was obtained by the author from reliable sources. However, while every effort has been make to ensure its accuracy, no responsibility for loss, damage or injury occasioned to any person acting or refraining from action as a result of information contained herein can be accepted by the publishers or author.

PasTest Revision Books and Intensive Courses
PasTest has been established in the field of postgraduate medical education since 1972, providing revision books and intensive study courses for doctors preparing for their professional examinations.

Books and courses are available for the following specialties:
MRCGP, MRCP Parts 1 and 2, MRCPCH Parts 1 and 2, MRCPsych, MRCS, MRCOG Parts 1 and 2, DRCOG, DCH, FRCA, Dentistry.

For further details contact:

PasTest, Freepost, Knutsford, Cheshire WA16 7BR
Tel: 01565 752000 Fax: 01565 650264
www.pastest.co.uk enquires@pastest.co.uk

Typeset by Saxon Graphics Ltd, Derby
Printed and bound in the UK by CPI Antony Rowe

Contents

List of contributors

Adam Feather FRCP
Senior Lecturer in Medical Education
Barts and The London Medical School,
Consultant Geriatrician, Newham University Hospital NHS Trust.

Charles H Knowles BChir PhD FRCS (Gen Surg)
Senior Lecturer and Hon Consultant Colorectal Surgeon
Centre for Academic Surgery
Royal London Hospital

Jonathan Round BA MBBS MRCP
Consultant Paediatric Intensivist - St George's Trust - London

Paola Domizio BSc MB BS FRCPath
Professor of Pathology Education
Barts and the London School of Medicine and Dentistry,
Queen Mary, University of London

Benjamin C T Field MBBS BMedSci MSc MRCP
MRC Clinical Research Training Fellow
Imperial College London, Hammersmith Hospital, London

John S P Lumley MS FRCS
Emeritus Professor of Vascular Surgery
St. Bartholomew's and the Royal London School of Medicine and Dentistry
Honorary Consultant Surgeon, St. Bartholomew's Hospital, London
Member of Council, Royal College of Surgeons and England

Preface

The problems of matching a medical examination to a training programme are compounded when the candidates being assessed have been trained in different programmes and might even be from different continents, with varying linguistic skills. Nevertheless, standard-setting bodies have a responsibility to examine at an appropriate level to ensure the delivery of optimal medical care to the community they represent. The purpose of the final examination should be to ensure the candidate's fitness to practise. Recent developments in examination systems have led to their division into their component parts, with an emphasis on the objective assessment of each section. Every qualifying doctor should therefore have proved competencies in written knowledge and clinical skills, and should be able to communicate, examine and relate to patients.

This text is devoted to the extended matching question (EMQ), a newer technique that is being used alongside (or replacing) the multiple choice question (MCQ). It has been used in North America since the mid-1990s, and after its introduction into the UK by the Royal College of General Practitioners in the MRCGP examination it has gained favour with a number of other Royal Colleges and medical schools.

There is always a danger that the technique is being examined as much as the medical information and whatever system is used, it is essential that the candidate is fully aware of, exposed to, and practised in the chosen technique for any examination. These three volumes of EMQs are intended to address this problem. They have been prepared for the final medical examination and the material is drawn from all parts of the undergraduate curriculum. They also serve as an introduction to EMQs for students who are in the early stages of their clinical course and provide suitable revision material for postgraduates entering this form of examination in every discipline. They will be helpful to examiners who are not versed in preparing EMQs, both from stylistic and content points of view. It is advisable to use teams of examiners and students to assess new questions, as opinions can vary on correct responses, especially those involving clinical management. The authors will not be surprised, or offended, if some of their own responses are challenged over time. In general, EMQs are more focused than MCQs and they are a welcome extension of this style of examination.

Introduction

We have included several innovations within these new editions. The most striking are the inclusion of radiology and other images, and the increased use of 'two step' items. Radiological images will help students remember both 'cause' and 'effect'. As with all data interpretation, one needs to be careful to treat the patient in conjunction with the radiological findings and not one in isolation of the other.

Traditional final and postgraduate examinations consisted of a written essay paper, a clinical examination consisting of long and short cases, and a viva. Although these methods provided excellent doctors for most of the last century, when they were assessed by objective measurements their reliability, reproducibility and validity came into question. Another problem with each of these methods was the limited amount of a curriculum that could be assessed in a single diet of an examination. It could therefore be a lottery as to whether candidates were asked questions on well-known or unfamiliar material or whether examiners were just asking for obscure details of their own specialty.

Continuous assessment of a course ensures matching of the training and assessment of its content. However, this is only possible for internal examinations.

Many techniques have been introduced to extend the area covered by a single examination and to standardise its marking system. The objective structured clinical examination (OSCE) has so far proved to be the most reproducible and reliable of the new systems. The written paper has received a great deal of attention: although the traditional free-response essay allows a candidate to demonstrate extensive knowledge, it covers an extremely small area of the course. When questions are set around the core of the curriculum, as is appropriate in a valid and reliable examination, these questions are easily spotted. Also, poor organisation of facts and illegible handwriting can contribute to failure as much as a lack of basic knowledge. Short answer and short-essay questions widen the area of assessment, and also reduce the reliance on technique. The MCQ has retained an important place in medical examinations for 30 years. The technique allows examination across a wide field, but clinical options are rarely totally right or wrong and well-constructed questions, even when set by a group of examiners, can still mislead well-prepared candidates.

The extended matching question (EMQ) is able to cover a wide area of the curriculum and assess the candidate's knowledge of clinically relevant information. It also goes beyond a simple recall of factual information, and assesses a candidate's ability to interpret data drawn from realistic, often existing, clinical problems.

Each EMQ in these books has a theme, a list of options, an introductory statement and a series of stems or scenarios. A quick look at any of the subsequent questions will provide an idea of its format. The chosen themes cover a wide range of topics that are all relevant and important in clinical practice. They include the anatomy of tissues and organs, symptoms, abnormal signs, normal and abnormal investigations, and specific diseases. They are organised by system and are listed in the contents at the beginning of each volume.

All options are feasible answers and are clustered around the chosen theme. They usually provide an extensive cover of the topic, and serve as revision aids, but are not necessarily all-inclusive. The larger the number of options, the less likely a correct answer can be obtained by chance, elimination or exclusion. However, the number also relates to the topic, the design of the question and the maximum number of feasible alternatives. Rare conditions are occasionally included, both as options and correct answers, providing a broad exposure to the field. There are 8–12 options for each theme, although the range can be extended to 5–20, depending on the topic. The options are listed alphabetically, unless amore appropriate order exists.

The introductory statement must be read carefully because it tells the reader what is expected of them. Usually, one option has to be chosen to answer each stem or scenario. The stems or scenarios determine the standard of a question, and must be pitched at the appropriate level for any examination. At an undergraduate level, scenarios are rich in uninterpreted symptoms, signs and investigations, but in more advanced examinations a clinical summary might be given without the need to sort out basic information. Key diagnostic criteria might be deliberately excluded in order to avoid making an answer too easy, or to stimulate the reader to think more deeply around a topic.

The scenarios must be sufficiently detailed that they only match the intended option from the list. However, in a few cases, where this increases understanding and clinical reasoning, more than one option has been identified: this is stated clearly within the introductory statement. Options provide a whole range of alternatives, including isolated facts, encouraging recognition and recall, but emphasis is given to clinical decision-making and interpretation of material, focusing on clinical scenarios. There are usually five scenarios per theme, but the number varies in different sections.

In the past, most EMQ vignettes required the students to derive an answer that was one of the items included in the alphabetical list. A two step item differs in that it requires the student to derive a fact or series of facts from the vignette (step one), and then link this with the items and theme of the vignette (step two). For example in a series where the theme is ECG rhythm strips (so all the items are rhythm strips) the first vignette implies that the patient is in fast AF. The student must be able to make the first answer of fast AF (first step) and then recognise the correct rhythm strip (second step). This two step approach is now commonly used in the later stages of the medical curriculum, to assess clinical diagnostic reasoning rather than straightforward factual recall.

The second half of each book gives the answers to each question, together with an extended explanation, providing an overview of the topic and a revision aid for each theme. It is not necessarily comprehensive, but should identify gaps and direct further reading.

The time allowed for an EMQ examination differs from that of an MCQ examination because each scenario can be quite complex, reflecting clinical practice, and time is needed to consider all options. In general, 120–160 scenarios can be answered in 2 hours, and not more than 200 should be included in a 3-hour examination. The scoring is 1 mark for each correct answer: if more than one option is correct, a mark or a proportion of the mark can be scored. There is no negative marking in EMQ assessment.

Ten practice examinations are listed at the end of the answer section of the book, drawing questions from across the syllabus: each is intended as a 2-hour examination.

Glossary

αFP	Alpha-fetoprotein
AAFB	Acid- and alcohol-fast bacilli
ABPI	Ankle–brachial pressure index
ACE	Angiotensin-converting enzyme
ACTH	Adrenocorticotrophic hormone
ADH	Antidiuretic hormone
AIDS	Acquired immunodeficiency syndrome
AIHA	Autoimmune haemolytic anaemia
ALL	Acute lymphoblastic leukaemia
ALT	Alanine aminotransferase
AMA	Antimitochondrial antibody
AML	Acute myeloid leukaemia
AMTS	Abridged mental test score
ANA	Antinuclear antibody
ANCA	Antineutrophil cytoplasmic antibody
APCKD	Adult polycystic kidney disease
APTT	Activated partial thromboplastin time
ASD	Atrial septal defect
ASOT	Antistreptolysin-O titre
AST	Aspartate aminotransferase
AV	Atrioventricular
AVSD	Atrioventricular septal defect
βhCG	Beta-human chorionic gonadotrophin
BMI	Body mass index
BMR	Best motor response
BP	Blood pressure
BPH	Benign prostatic hypertrophy
bpm	beats per minute
BVR	Best vocal response
c-ANCA	cytoplasmic ANCA
CIN	Cervical intraepithelial neoplasia
CLL	Chronic lymphocytic leukaemia
CLO	*Campylobacter*-like organism
CML	Chronic myeloid leukaemia

CMV	Cytomegalovirus
CNS	Central nervous system
COPD	Chronic obstructive pulmonary disease
COX	Cyclo-oxygenase
CREST	Calcinosis, Raynaud's, oesophageal dysmotility, sclerodactyly and telangiectasia
CRF	Chronic renal failure
CRH	Corticotrophin-releasing hormone
CRP	C-reactive protein
CSF	Cerebrospinal fluid
CT	Computed tomography
CVP	Central venous pressure
DC	Direct current
DDAVP®	Des-amino-D-arginine vasopressin
DIC	Disseminated intravascular coagulation
DMARD	Disease-modifying agents of rheumatoid disease
DNA	Deoxyribonucleic acid
dsDNA	Double-stranded DNA
DVT	Deep venous thrombosis
EBV	Epstein–Barr virus
ECG	Electrocardiography (or -gram)
EEG	Electroencephalography (or -gram
EMG	Electromyelography (or –gram)
EMU	Early-morning urine
ENA	Extractable nuclear antigen
ERCP	Endoscopic retrograde cholangiopancreatography
ESR	Erythrocyte sedimentation rate
ESRF	End-stage renal failure
Fab	Fragment antigen binding
FAP	Familial adenomatous polyposis
FBC	Full blood count
Fc	Fragment crystallisable
FEV_1	Forced expiratory volume in 1 second
FNAC	Fine-needle aspiration cytology
FSH	Follicle-stimulating hormone
fT_3	Tri-iodo-thyronine
fT_4	Free thyroxine
FTA	Fluorescent *Treponema* absorption
FVC	Vital capacity during forced expiration
G6PD	Glucose-6-phosphate dehydrogenase
γGT	Gamma-glutamyltransferase
GCA	Giant-cell arteritis
GCS	Glasgow coma scale
GCSF	Granulocyte colony-stimulating factor
GnRH	Gonadotrophin-releasing hormone
GORD	Gastro-oesophageal reflux disease
GP	General Practitioner
GVHD	Graft-versus-host disease
$Hb\,A_{1c}$	Glycosylated haemoglobin
HBV	Hepatitis B virus
hCG	Human chorionic gonadotrophin

HDL	High-density lipoprotein
HHV	Human herpesvirus
HIV	Human immunodeficiency virus
HLA	Human leucocyte antigen
HMGCoA	Hydroxymethyl glutaryl co-enzyme A
HNPCC	Hereditary non-polyposis colorectal cancer (syndrome)
HOCM	Hypertrophic obstructive cardiomyopathy
HONK	Hyperosmolar non-ketotic acidosis
HPV	Human papillomavirus
HSMN	Hereditary sensory and motor neuropathy
HSP	Henoch–Schönlein purpura
IAPP	Islet amyloid polypeptide
IBD	Inflammatory bowel disease
IBS	Irritable bowel syndrome
IDDM	Insulin-dependent diabetes mellitus
Ig	Immunoglobulin
IGT	Impaired glucose tolerance
IHD	Ischaemic heart disease
IL1	Interleukin 1
INO	Internuclear ophthalmoplegia
INR	International normalised ratio
IVU	Intravenous urography/gram
IVP	Intravenous pyelography/gram
JVP	Jugular venous pressure
LDH	Lactate dehydrogenase
LDL	Low-density lipoprotein
LEMS	Lambert–Eaton myasthenic syndrome
LFT	Liver function test
LH	Luteinising hormone
LKM	Liver, kidney-microsomal
LVF	Left ventricular failure
LVH	Left ventricular hypertrophy
MALT	Mucosa-associated lymphoid tissue
MCHC	Mean corpuscular haemoglobin concentration
MCV	Mean corpuscular volume
MEN	Multiple endocrine neoplasia
MGUS	Monoclonal gammapathy of unknown significance
MHC	Major histocompatibility complex
MI	Myocardial infarction
MIBG	Metaiodobenzylguanidine
MLF	Medial longitudinal fasciculus
MND	Motor neurone disease
MODS	Multiorgan dysfunction syndrome
MRI	Magnetic resonance imaging
MSU	Mid-stream urine
NADPH	Nicotinamide adenine dinucleotide phosphate
NEP	Nucleotide excision pathway
NK	Natural killer (cell)
NSAID	Non-steroidal anti-inflammatory drug
OGD	Oesophagastroduodenoscopy
OGTT	Oral glucose tolerance test

PAN	Polyarteritis nodosa
p-ANCA	perinuclear ANCA
PAS	Periodic acid–Schiff
PBC	Primary biliary cirrhosis
PCKD	Polycystic kidney disease
PCOS	Polycystic ovary syndrome
PCR	Polymerase chain reaction
PCV	Packed cell volume
PDA	Patent ductus arteriosus
PEA	Pulseless electrical activity
PID	Pelvic inflammatory disease
PLE	Protein-losing enteropathy
PND	Paroxysmal nocturnal dyspnoea
PSA	Prostate-specific antigen
PT	Prothrombin time
PTH	Parathyroid hormone
PTT	Partial thromboplastin time
PUO	Pyrexia of unknown origin
RNA	Ribonucleic acidt
rT_3	Reverse tri-iodothyronine
RTA	Road traffic accident
SACD	Subacute combined degeneration of the cord
SARS	Severe acute respiratory syndrome
SCBU	Special Care Baby Unit
SHBG	Sex hormone-binding globulin
SIADH	Syndrome of inappropriate ADH secretion
SIRS	Systemic inflammatory response syndrome
SLE	Systemic lupus erythematosus
SSRI	Selective serotonin reuptake inhibitor
TB	Tuberculosis
TMRP	Transmembrane regulator protein
TNF-α	Tumour necrosis factor alpha
TPHA	*Treponema pallidum* haemagglutination assay
TSH	Thyroid-stimulating hormone
TT	Thrombin time
TURP	Transurethral resection of the prostate
U&Es	Urea and electrolytes
UTI	Urinary tract infection
UV	Ultraviolet
VDRL	Venereal Disease Research Laboratory
VER	Visual-evoked response
VMA	Vanillyl mandelic acid
V/Q	Ventilation-perfusion (scan)
VSD	Ventricular septal defect
vWF	von Willebrand factor
WCC	White cell count
WHO	World Health Organisation

Normal values

Blood, serum and plasma

Haematology
Haemoglobin
    Males   13.5–17.5 g/dl
    Females   11.5–15.5 g/dl
MCV   76–98 fl
Haematocrit   0.35–0.55
WCC $4\text{–}11 \times 10^9/l$
    Neutrophils $2.5\text{–}7.58 \times 10^9/l$
    Lymphocytes $1.5\text{–}3.5 \times 10^9/l$
Platelets $150\text{–}400 \times 10^9/l$

ESR   0–10 mm in the 1st hour

PT   10.6–14.9 s
PTT   23.0–35.0 s
TT   10.5–15.5 s
Fibrinogen   125–300 mg/dl

Vitamin B_{12} 160–900 pmol/l
Folate   1.5–10.0 mg/l
Ferritin
    Males   20–250 µg/l
    Females   10–120 µg/l

Immunoglobulins
IgM   0.5–2.0 g/l
IgG   5–16 g/l
IgA   1.0–4.0 g/l

Biochemistry

Na^+	135–145 mmol/l
K^+	3.5–5.0 mmol/l
Urea	2.5–6.5 mmol/l
Creatinine	50–120 μmol/l
ALT	5–30 IU/l
AST	10–40 IU/l
Bilirubin	2–17 μmol/l
Alkaline phosphatase	30–130 IU/l
Albumin	35–55 g/l
γGT	5–30 IU/l
αFP	<10 kU/l
Corrrected Ca^{2+}	2.20–2.60 mmol/l
PO_4^{3-}	0.70–1.40 mmol/l
Creatine kinase	23–175 IU/l
LDH	100–190 IU/l
Amylase	<200 U/l
Lactate	0.5–2.2 mmol/l
Mg^{2+}	0.75–1.00 mmol/l
Urate	0.1–0.4 mmol/l
CRP	0–10 mg/l
Troponin	<0.1 ng/ml

Diabetes

Glucose	
Random	3.5–5.5 mmol/l*
Fasting	<7 mmol/l
Hb A_{1c}	<7.0%

* If >5.5 mmol/l, then OGTT at 2 hours:
   <7.8 mmol/l = normal
   7.8–11.0 = IGT
   >11.1 mmol/l = diabetes mellitus

Endocrinology

TSH	0.17–3.2 μU/l
fT_4	11–22 pmol/l
fT_3	3.5–5 pmol/l
Cortisol	
9 am	140–500 nmol/l
Midnight	50–300 nmol/l
Growth hormone	<10 ng/ml
Cholesterol	<5.2 mmol/l
Triglycerides	0–1.5 mmol/l
LDL	<3.5 mmol/l
HDL	>1.0 mmol/l
Total/HDL	<5.0 mmol/l
FSH	1–25 U/l
LH	1–70 U/l
Prolactin	<400 mU/l

Blood gases

pH	7.35–7.45
$PaCO_2$	4.6–6.0 kPa
PaO_2	10.5–13.5 kPa
HCO_3^-	24–30 mmol/l
Base excess	–2 to +2.0 mmol/l

CSF

Protein	<0.45 g/l
Glucose	2.5–3.9 mmol/l (two-thirds plasma value)
Cells	<5/mm^3 (WCC)
Opening pressure	6–20 cmH$_2$O

QUESTIONS

CHAPTER **1**

Gastroenterology

1. THEME: ANATOMY OF THE ALIMENTARY TRACT

A   Appendix
B   Ascending colon
C   Duodenojejunal flexure
D   Ileocaecal valve
E   Jejunum
F   Oesophagogastric junction
G   Pylorus
H   Second part of the duodenum
I   Sigmoid colon mesentery
J   Splenic flexure of the colon

For each of the statements below, select the most appropriate segment of gut from the above list. Each segment may be used once, more than once or not at all.

1.   Contains mucous glands whose coiled pits extend into the submucosa.

2.   Lies to the right of the midline, at the level of the upper border of the first lumbar vertebra.

3.   Overlies the left ureter.

4.   Overlies the lower pole of the right kidney.

5.   Has mucosa characterised by prominent villi.

2. THEME: VOMITING

A   Acute abdomen
B   Central nervous system causes
C   Drug therapy
D   Gastroenteritis due to *Bacillus cereus*
E   Gastroenteritis due to *Salmonella* spp.
F   Gastroenteritis due to *Staphylococcus aureus*
G   Gastric outflow obstruction
H   Large-intestinal obstruction
I   Small-intestinal obstruction
J   Uraemia

The patients below have all presented with vomiting. Please select the most appropriate cause from the above list. Each cause may be used once, more than once or not at all.

1. An 80-year-old woman is accompanied by her daughter to the Emergency Department. She gives a 2-day history of nausea and vomiting and is slightly confused. Her past medical history includes atrial fibrillation, osteoarthritis and recently diagnosed hypertension. She was started on a low-dose bendroflumethiazide 3 weeks ago by her GP. She claims to have been compliant with her medications, which include digoxin and co-dydramol. On examination, her temperature is 36.8 °C, her pulse is 56 beats per minute (bpm), irregularly irregular and her blood pressure (BP) is 145/85 mmHg. There is mild epigastric tenderness. Her urea and electrolytes (U&Es) are: Na^+ 138 mmol/l, K^+ 3.1 mmol/l, urea 8.6 mmol/l, creatinine 142 μmol/l. □

2. A 25-year-old student gives an 8-hour history of frequent vomiting, being 'unable to keep anything down'. He also has some cramp-like abdominal pain. On general examination he appears pale and clammy and is shivering; abdominal examination is unremarkable. There is no previous medical history or drug history. Investigations show: haemoglobin 14.7 g/dl, white cell count (WCC) 11.8 × 10⁹/l, platelets 368 × 10⁹/l; Na^+ 135 mmol/l, K^+ 3.4 mmol/l, urea 7.7 mmol/l, creatinine 70 μmol/l. □

3. A 4-week-old baby is admitted with a 4-day history of projectile vomiting of large amounts of curdled milk shortly after every feed. This pattern is observed in hospital and a 2-cm, palpable mass is felt on palpation in the epigastric region during feeding. Investigations show: haemoglobin 17.0 g/dl, WCC 4.6 × 10⁹/l, platelets 170 × 10⁹/l; Na^+ 131 mmol/l, K^+ 2.9 mmol/l, urea 7.5 mmol/l, creatinine 43 μmol/l. □

4. A 22-year-old woman presents with a 3-day history of colicky, central abdominal pain and vomiting. The pain is partially relieved by vomiting and the vomitus is described as dark-green. On examination, she is dehydrated and the abdomen is distended but non-tender to palpation. She has previously had an appendectomy for appendicitis that was complicated by peritonitis. Investigations show: haemoglobin 10.6 g/dl, WCC 11.1 × 10⁹/l, platelets 454 × 10⁹/l; Na^+ 130 mmol/l, K^+ 3.3 mmol/l, urea 10.0 mmol/l, creatinine 100 μmol/l. □

5. A 12-year-old boy presents with a 12-hour history of abdominal pain, nausea and vomiting. On examination, he is febrile (38.8 °C), tachycardic, and has tenderness and guarding in the right iliac fossa. The full blood count (FBC) shows: haemoglobin 13.6 g/dl, WCC 14.1 × 10⁹/l, platelets 325 × 10⁹/l.

3. THEME: HAEMATEMESIS

A   Gastric carcinoma
B   Gastric erosions
C   Gastric leiomyoma
D   Hiatus hernia
E   Oesophagitis
F   Oesophageal carcinoma
G   Oesophageal varices
H   Mallory–Weiss tear
I   Peptic ulcer disease (duodenal/gastric ulcer)
J   Zollinger–Ellison syndrome

The patients below have all presented with haematemesis. Please select the most appropriate diagnosis from the above list. Each diagnosis may be used once, more than once or not at all.

1. A 70-year-old man is admitted to a burns unit with 40% burns to the body. He is sedated, given opioid analgesia and started on prophylactic antibiotics in addition to vigorous fluid resuscitation and dressings. The following day he has several episodes of haematemesis. Tests show: haemoglobin 9.2 g/dl, WCC 15.1 × 10^9/l, platelets 410 × 10^9/l; international normalised ratio (INR) 1.0.

2. A 32-year-old woman who has been investigated for 1 year for recurrent peptic ulceration is admitted with haematemesis. Ranitidine had previously failed to control her symptoms and she is presently taking omeprazole 40 mg. Endoscopy reveals a 2-cm, actively bleeding ulcer in the duodenum. A computed tomographic (CT) scan shows a 2-cm mass in the pancreas.

3. A 45-year-old man is brought into the Emergency Department after several episodes of vomiting of fresh blood. The patient is drowsy and little other history is available. Investigations show: haemoglobin 8.1 g/dl, mean corpuscular volume (MCV) 106 fl, platelets 167 × 10^9/l, WCC 11.7 × 10^9/l with platelets 167 × 10^9/l; INR 2.1.

4. A 73-year-old man presents with several episodes of coffee-ground vomiting. Further questioning reveals a 5-month history of epigastric discomfort, nausea, anorexia (with inability to eat normal-sized meals) and weight loss. The FBC shows: haemoglobin 7.9 g/dl, MCV 76.6 fl, WCC 5.3 × 10^9/l, platelets 333 × 10^9/l, and the INR is 1.1.

5. A 22-year-old medical student comes in to the Emergency Department after the annual college 'beer race'. After vomiting several times he notices bright - blood in the vomitus. He had only consumed 12 pints of beer (as is the custom to complete the race). The FBC shows: haemoglobin 14.2 g/dl, MCV 85.6 fl, WCC 8.2 × 10^9/l, platelets 450 × 10^9/l, and his INR is 1.0.

4. THEME: CONSTIPATION

A   Carcinoma of the colon/rectum
B   Chronic idiopathic constipation
C   Depression
D   Diabetes mellitus
E   Diverticular disease
F   Hypercalcaemia
G   Hypothyroidism
H   Iatrogenic (drug therapy)
I   Pelvic nerve or spinal cord injury
J   Simple constipation

The patients below have all presented with constipation. Please select the most appropriate diagnosis from the above list. Each cause may be used once, more than once or not at all.

1. A 66-year-old man presents with a 3-month history of difficulty passing stool. On direct questioning, his bowels had previously been open daily with the passage of normal, formed stool. He now complains of straining to pass small, worm-like stools with mucus. He also has a sensation of needing to pass stool but being unable to do so.

2. A 28-year-old woman with a history of chronic schizophrenia is referred by the psychiatric team after complaining of abdominal pain, bloating and constipation. She opens her bowels approximately twice a week with the passage of hard stool. She also complains of a dry mouth.

3. A 92-year-old woman falls and fractures her right neck of femur. She has been admitted to hospital by the orthopaedic team under whom she has a dynamic hip screw. Six days post-operatively she is complaining of colicky lower abdominal pain and the nurses tell you that she has not opened her bowels since the operation. Faeces are palpable in the left colon and on rectal examination. A plain abdominal radiograph confirms the presence of faecal loading

4. A 24-year-old girl gives a lifelong history of constipation from early childhood. She opens her bowels every 2 weeks and has little or no urge to pass faeces between these times. She complains of chronic lower abdominal discomfort, nausea and bloating.

5. A 56-year-old man is admitted to hospital with a short history of lower abdominal pain and difficulty opening his bowels. At the time of admission he has not passed faeces for 6 days and is now experiencing difficulties passing urine (hesitancy, poor stream). Direct questioning reveals that he has a 6-month history of chronic cough with occasional hemoptysis, which he puts down to his being a smoker. His wife thinks that he might also have lost some weight recently.

5. THEME: DIARRHOEA

A   Amoebic dysentery
B   Autonomic neuropathy
C   Bacterial enterocolitis
D   Caecal carcinoma
E   Crohn's disease
F   Irritable bowel syndrome
G   Overflow (faecal impaction)
H   Pseudomembranous colitis
I   Thyrotoxicosis
J   Ulcerative colitis

The patients below have all presented with diarrhoea as a predominant symptom. Please select the most appropriate diagnosis from the above list. Each diagnosis may be used once, more than once or not at all.

1. A 25-year-old man has returned recently from a holiday in Mexico. He gives a 24-hour history of severe, cramp-like, lower abdominal pain with passage of watery, brown, offensive diarrhoea. He had felt generally unwell, with flu-like symptoms for the preceding 2–3 days. On examination, he is clinically dehydrated and febrile (38.2 °C) with a pulse of 100 bpm. His haemoglobin is 15.4 g/dl and his WCC is 14.8 × 10^9/1.

2. A 70-year-old man presents with a history of several months of diarrhoea. He previously opened his bowels once daily with formed stool. He has lost approximately 1 stone in weight. Investigations show: haemoglobin 8.1 g/dl, MCV 72.2 fl, WCC 7.6 × 10^9/l; erythrocyte sedimentation rate (ESR) 40 mm/h; C-reactive protein (CRP) 55 mg/l.

3. A 32-year-old woman presents with a 2-week history of passing bloody diarrhoea with mucus up to 12 times per day. This is associated with lower abdominal, cramp-like pain and general malaise. On examination, she looks pale and generally unwell and there is some tenderness in the left-iliac fossa. Investigations show: haemoglobin 9.8 g/dl; MCV 76.2 fl; WCC 12.2 × 10^9/1; ESR 100 mm/h; CRP 123 mg/l.

4. A 24-year-old woman gives a long history (several years) of intermittent diarrhoea and constipation. She also complains of abdominal bloating and left iliac fossa pain. The pain and bloating are made worse by eating and are relieved to some extent by defecation. Abdominal examination is unremarkable, and investigations show: haemoglobin 12.6 g/dl, WCC 6.5 × 10^9/l; ESR 10 mm/h; CRP 5 mg/l. Flexible sigmoidoscopy is normal.

5. An 80-year-old woman is admitted to hospital with a left lower lobe pneumonia. She receives intravenous amoxicillin and cefuroxime. You are asked to review her because the nurses are having difficulty coping with her frequent episodes of diarrhoea and incontinence. Rectal examination reveals an empty rectum.

6. THEME: WEIGHT LOSS

A   Alcohol dependency
B   Anorexia nervosa
C   Carcinomatosis
D   Cardiac failure
E   Coeliac disease
F   Crohn's disease
G   Giardiasis
H   Thyrotoxicosis
I   Tuberculosis
J   Type 1 diabetes mellitus

The following patients have all presented with weight loss. Please choose the most appropriate diagnosis from the above list. Each diagnosis may be used once, more than once or not at all.

1. A 22-year-old woman with hypopigmented patches over the dorsum of her hands presents to her GP with weight loss, loose stools and oligomenorrhoea. On examination, she has onycholysis, fine tremor, resting tachycardia and warm peripheries.

2. A 16-year-old schoolboy presents to his GP with a 6-week history of malaise, weight loss and polydipsia. Examination is unremarkable other than his obvious weight loss. Initial investigations reveal: haemoglobin 14.4 g/dl, MCV 82 fl, WCC 7.2 × 10⁹/l, platelets 229 × 10⁹/l; Na⁺ 135 mmol/l, K⁺ 4.1 mmol/l, urea 4.1 mmol/l, creatinine 76 μmol/l; random blood glucose 18.9 mmol/l; thyroid-stimulating hormone (TSH) 1.43 mU/l, free thyroxine (fT_4) 22.6 pmol/l.

3. A 41-year-old woman presents to her GP with weight loss and 'anxiety'. She confesses to feeling low since her divorce some 18 months ago. On examination she is thin and mildly icteric. Cardiovascular and respiratory examinations are unremarkable but abdominal examination reveals 3-cm hepatomegaly below the right costal margin. Investigations reveal: haemoglobin 9.4 g/dl, MCV 101 fl, WCC 4.2 × 10⁹/l, platelets 107 × 10⁹/l; Na⁺ 131 mmol/l, K⁺ 4.1 mmol/l, urea 2.1 mmol/l, creatinine 76 μmol/l; random blood glucose 3.9 mmol/l; total bilirubin 27 μmol/l, aspartate aminotransferase (AST) 76 IU/l, alanine aminotransferase (ALT) 59 IU/l, alkaline phosphatase 133 IU/l, albumin 31 g/l; INR 1.3.

4. A 51-year-old woman presents to her GP with weight loss, anorexia and swelling of the abdomen. On examination she is unwell, thin and pale, and has signs of a left pleural effusion, hepatomegaly and shifting dullness in the abdomen. Her chest radiograph confirms the effusion and shows multiple opacities in both lung fields.

5. A 24-year-old man returns from Nepal with a 6-week history of fever, bloody diarrhoea, the passage of mucus and weight loss. On examination, he is clinically anaemic, has aphthous ulceration of the mouth and mild tenderness of the abdomen. Sigmoidoscopy shows mucosal ulceration and biopsy confirms 'superficial ulceration with chronic inflammatory infiltrate within the lamina propria, goblet cell depletion and crypt abscesses'. Stool culture and microscopy are unremarkable.

7. THEME: ABDOMINAL PAIN I

A   Acute pancreatitis
B   Appendicitis
C   Ascending cholangitis
D   Cholecystitis
E   Diverticulitis
F   Faecal peritonitis
G   Gastritis
H   Large-bowel obstruction
I   Peptic ulcer disease
J   Ureteric colic

The patients below have all presented with abdominal pain. Please select the most appropriate diagnosis from the above list. Each diagnosis may be used once, more than once or not at all.

1. A 60-year-old man presents with fever (39.2 °C), rigors and upper abdominal pain. On examination, he is clinically jaundiced and has a systolic blood pressure of 90 mmHg.

2. A 17-year-old boy with no previous medical history presents with a 24-hour history of increasing right iliac fossa pain associated with nausea and vomiting. The urine is clear. A FBC shows a haemoglobin of 12.5 g/dl and a WCC of 16.8×10^9/l.

3. A 38-year-old man with a history of attending the Emergency Department with injuries sustained while drunk presents with a 2-day history of increasing epigastric and left-sided upper abdominal pain radiating to the back. He is retching continuously in the Department and is clinically dehydrated. He is found to have ketones and a trace of glucose in the urine. Blood investigations show: WCC 14.2×10^9/l, MCV 104 fl; Na$^+$ 135 mmol/l, K$^+$ 3.2 mmol/l, urea 10.1 mmol/l.

4. A 73-year-old woman presents with a long history of intermittent left iliac fossa pain and constipation. In the last few days this has become more severe and she has felt nauseous and unable to eat. Examination reveals tenderness and guarding in the left iliac fossa. Urine dipstick testing shows a trace of blood. An FBC shows: haemoglobin 12.7 g/dl, WCC 15.3×10^9/l.

5. A 45-year-old Turkish man presents with a short history of severe, right-sided abdominal pain that is radiating to the groin. He is writhing around, unable to sit or lie still. No other history is available. An abdominal radiograph is normal. The only investigation that comes back positive is the finding of some blood in the urine.

8. THEME: ABDOMINAL PAIN II

A   Diabetes mellitus
B   Dissecting aortic aneurysm
C   Large-bowel obstruction
D   Myocardial infarction
E   Oesophageal reflux disease
F   Perforated diverticular disease
G   Perforated duodenal ulcer
H   Ruptured abdominal aortic aneurysm
I   Sickle-cell disease
J   Small-bowel obstruction

The patients below have all presented with abdominal pain. Please select the most appropriate diagnosis from the above list. Each diagnosis may be used once, more than once or not at all.

1.   A 92-year-old man presents with a 1-day history of upper abdominal pain and nausea. On general examination he is sweaty and breathless. He has no gastrointestinal symptoms and a normal abdominal examination. Investigations reveal: haemoglobin 11.2 g/dl, WCC 10.8 × 10⁹/1; troponin I 20.6 IU/l, creatine kinase 2000 IU/l.

2.   A 36-year-old woman who underwent an operation for perforated appendix 1 year ago presents with a 3-day history of increasing, central, colicky abdominal pain. She has been vomiting today and feels distended. She opened her bowels normally yesterday. Investigations reveal: haemoglobin 13.2 g/dl, WCC 9.8 × 10⁹/l; K⁺ 3.4 mmol/l.

3.   A 72-year-old man, who is a known hypertensive, presents with sudden-onset (30 minutes ago), very severe epigastric pain radiating to the back. On examination he is shocked, with a pulse of 120 bpm and BP of 90/55 mmHg. The femoral pulses are present but weak. There is generalised abdominal tenderness and guarding.

4.   A 76-year-old woman presents with a 3-day history of intermittent lower abdominal pain. She has not opened her bowels or passed wind for 2 days and has noticed that she has become very distended today. Abdominal examination reveals a distended, hyper-resonant but non-tender abdomen.

5.   A 40-year-old man presents with a rapid onset of severe, constant epigastric pain. On examination, he is lying still and appears very distressed, pulse 118 bpm, BP 120/70 mmHg, respiratory rate 30/minute. The abdomen is tender and there is intense guarding with rigidity. The abdomen is silent to auscultation.

9. THEME: ABDOMINAL MASS

A Appendix mass
B Carcinoma of the head of the pancreas
C Carcinoma of the kidney
D Carcinoma of the sigmoid colon
E Carcinoma of the stomach
F Cirrhosis of the liver
G Diverticular mass
H Gallstone disease
I Pancreatic pseudocyst
J Splenomegaly

The patients below have all presented with a palpable abdominal mass. Please select the most appropriate diagnosis from the above list. Each diagnosis may be used once, more than once or not at all.

1. A 35-year-old alcoholic presents with a 1-month history of epigastric pain, fullness and nausea. He has previously had two or three episodes of severe epigastric pain associated with vomiting. Examination reveals a large, slightly tender, rather indistinct mass in the upper abdomen with no other specific features.

2. A 56-year-old woman presents with a 2-week history of increasing jaundice and pruritus. Direct questioning reveals that over the past few months she has had some upper abdominal pain, radiating to the left side of the back, and has lost approximately 10 kg in weight. A smooth hemi-ovoid mass is palpable in the right upper quadrant which moves with respiration. It is dull to percussion.

3. A 53-year-old man presents with a 10-day history of increasing jaundice and pruritus. Direct questioning reveals that he has become increasingly constipated over the past year with some loss of appetite and weight. Examination reveals a large, hard, irregular mass in the right upper quadrant and epigastrium which moves on respiration and is dull to percussion, and a further mass in the left iliac fossa.

4. A 58-year-old woman presents with an acute haematemesis. On examination she is slightly jaundiced and confused. The abdomen is generally distended with shifting dullness. A large mass is palpable in the right upper quadrant and epigastrium which moves on respiration and is dull to percussion.

5. A 46-year-old woman presents with a 5-day history of severe right upper quadrant pain, nausea and vomiting. On examination, she is febrile and a very tender mass is palpable in the right upper quadrant that moves with respiration and is dull to percussion. She is not jaundiced.

10. THEME: DYSPHAGIA

A   Achalasia
B   Bulbar palsy
C   Chagas' disease
D   Gastro-oesophageal reflux disease
E   Myasthenia gravis
F   Oesophageal candidiasis
G   Oesophageal carcinoma
H   Pharyngeal pouch
I   Pharyngeal web
J   Pseudobulbar palsy
K   Scleroderma

The patients below have all presented with difficulty swallowing (dysphagia). Please select the most appropriate diagnosis from the above list. Each diagnosis may be used once, more than once or not at all.

1. A 72-year-old man presents with a 6-month history of progressive difficulty swallowing. He is now only able to swallow small quantities of fluids and has lost 10 kg in weight. Examination is unremarkable apart from his wasted appearance. Liver function tests (LFTs) show: bilirubin 20 μmol/l, total protein 58 g/l, albumin 28 g/l, alkaline phosphatase 96 IU/l.

2. A 45-year-old man presents with a 6-month history of progressive difficulty with speech and swallowing. On examination, there is some weakness of facial muscles bilaterally, with drooling. The tongue is flaccid and shows fasciculation and the jaw jerk is absent. Eye movements are normal.

3. A 50-year-old woman presents with a history of chest pain associated with regurgitation of solids and liquids equally, both occurring shortly after swallowing. Radiological investigation reveals a dilated oesophagus with a tapering lower oesophageal segment. Oesophageal manometry demonstrates failure of relaxation of the lower oesophageal sphincter.

4. A 26-year-old man who has undergone a renal transplant presents with a 3-day history of severe odynophagia and difficulty swallowing. Barium swallow and endoscopy demonstrate generalised ulceration of the oesophagus. His medications include oral prednisolone and ciclosporin.

5. A 30–year-old man presents with a long history of epigastric burning pain which is worse at night. He also suffers from severe burning pain in the chest when drinking hot liquids. Recently he has noted some difficulty swallowing solids. Endoscopy reveals confluent circumferential erosions and stricturing in the lower oesophagus. Twenty-four-hour ambulatory oesophageal pH measurement demonstrates a pH of <4 for 10% of the recording.

11. THEME: DISEASES OF THE STOMACH

A   Active chronic gastritis
B   Acute erosive gastritis
C   Adenocarcinoma
D   Adenoma
E   Carcinoid tumour
F   Chronic peptic ulcer
G   Gastrointestinal stromal tumour
H   Kaposi's sarcoma
I   Lymphoma of mucosa-associated lymphoid tissue (MALT)
J   Ménétrier's disease
K   Pyloric stenosis
L   Reflux gastropathy

For each of the patients below, select the gastric disease that they are most likely to have from the above list. Each disease may be used once, more than once or not at all.

1. A 63-year-old woman presents with a 2-month history of anorexia, weight loss and epigastric pain. Blood tests done by her GP reveal an iron-deficiency anaemia. Endoscopy shows a thickened and rigid gastric wall without an obvious mass lesion. Biopsies show numerous signet-ring cells diffusely infiltrating the mucosa.

2. A 42-year-old woman with rheumatoid arthritis presents with two episodes of melaena. She has recently started taking a new non-steroidal anti-inflammatory drug (NSAID). Endoscopy shows numerous superficial mucosal defects throughout the stomach, some of which are bleeding.

3. A 51-year-old man presents with a 3-month history of dyspepsia and weight loss. Endoscopy reveals thickened mucosal folds and a 2-cm antral ulcer. Biopsies show a heavy infiltrate of atypical lymphocytes with clusters of intraepithelial lymphocytes.

4. A 26-year-old, HIV-positive man presents with a 2-week history of dyspepsia and epigastric pain. Endoscopy shows a purple, plaque-like lesion in the fundus. Biopsies of the lesion show slit-like vascular spaces surrounded by proliferating spindle cells.

5. A 12-year-old man presents with a long history of epigastric discomfort related to meals. Endoscopy shows diffuse erythema in the antrum without obvious ulceration. Antral biopsies show an infiltrate of lymphocytes, plasma cells and neutrophils in the gastric mucosa. None of the lymphocytes are atypical. A special stain reveals numerous *Helicobacter pylori* organisms lining the mucosal surface.

6. A 52-year-old man presents with a 6-month history of burning epigastric pain that is relieved by antacids and food. He has recently had two episodes of vomiting coffee grounds. Endoscopy shows a 3-cm, punched-out ulcer in the antrum. Biopsies of the ulcer reveal inflammatory debris and granulation tissue only. Biopsies from adjacent mucosa show chronic inflammation with no evidence of neoplasia.

12. THEME: DYSPEPSIA AND PEPTIC ULCER DISEASE

A   Barrett's oesophagus
B   Biliary gastritis
C   Duodenal ulcer
D   Duodenitis
E   Gastric ulcer
F   Gastro-oesophageal reflux disease
G   Haemorrhagic gastritis
H   Oesophageal stricture
I   Pyloric stenosis
J   Zollinger–Ellison syndrome

The following patients have all presented with dyspepsia or complications of peptic ulcer disease. Please choose the most appropriate diagnosis from the above list. Each diagnosis may be used once, more than once or not at all.

1. A 54-year-old man presents in the Emergency Department with two episodes of fresh haematemesis over the preceding hour. On examination, he is pale but haemodynamically stable and well perfused. He has no lymphadenopathy or signs of chronic liver disease and the only significant finding is epigastric tenderness. Oesophagogastroduodenoscopy (OGD) confirms a lesion in the first part of the duodenum which requires injection. His *Campylobacter*-like organism (CLO) test is strongly positive.

2. A 59-year-old man presents to his GP with severe retrosternal burning pain. On examination, he is pale but otherwise well, with no significant findings. Upper gastrointestinal endoscopy reveals long-standing changes of gastro-oesophageal reflux and biopsy confirms 'metaplastic changes within the epithelium'.

3. A 34-year-old man with severe peptic ulcer disease is seen in the Emergency Department with epigastric pain and vomiting. On examination, he looks unwell and has severe vomiting. Abdominal examination reveals mild, generalised tenderness and a succussion splash. Initial investigations show: haemoglobin 10.9 g/dl, MCV 73 fl, WCC 10.9 × 10^9/l, platelets 342 × 10^9/l; Na$^+$ 135 mmol/l, K$^+$ 2.9 mmol/l, HCO$_3^-$ 48 mmol/l, urea 5.9 mmol/l, creatinine 95 μmol/l. An abdominal radiograph shows 'large gastric bubble, nil else'.

4. A 69-year-old woman with a long history of dyspepsia is seen by her GP with mid-thoracic dysphagia to solids associated with pain on food reaching the sticking point. Examination is unremarkable but routine investigations confirm a microcytic anaemia.

5. A 41-year-old man is referred to the Gastroenterology Out-patient Clinic with a 3-month history of worsening epigastric pain and dyspepsia. Upper (GI) endoscopy confirms multiple peptic ulcers in the stomach and duodenum, with ulceration in the lower oesophagus. His serum gastrin levels are grossly elevated.

13. THEME: TREATMENT OF DYSPEPSIA

A   Aluminium hydroxide
B   Bismuth
C   Calcium carbonate
D   Carbenoxolone
E   Cimetidine
F   Magnesium trisilicate
G   Misoprostol
H   Omeprazole
I   Ranitidine
J   Sucralfate

The following patients have all presented with side-effects of their dyspepsia treatment. Please choose the most appropriate drug from the above list. Each drug may be used once, more than once or not at all.

1. A 49-year-old woman is placed on prophylactic protection for her gastrointestinal tract after being started on a NSAID tablet for her rheumatoid arthritis. Two weeks later she returns with diarrhoea and vaginal bleeding, both of which resolve when the prophylaxis is changed.

2. A 76-year-old man is seen in the Out-patients' Department with long-standing dyspepsia for which his GP started him on therapy some 15 years ago. On examination, he is mildly anaemic, has no lymphadenopathy but has marked gynaecomastia. Examination is otherwise unremarkable.

3. A 31-year-old businessman is seen by his GP because of worsening constipation. During the last few months he has suffered with severe dyspepsia and has been drinking large amounts of an antacid preparation. Examination is unremarkable other than a loaded rectum.

4. A 46-year-old woman is seen in the Emergency Department with shortness of breath and a chest infection. The only medication she is taking is an over-the-counter preparation for heartburn. Her routine arterial blood gases reveal: pH 7.54, $PaCO_2$ 4.7 kPa, PaO_2 11.1 kPa, oxygen saturation 96%, HCO_3^- 36.7 mmol/l.

5. A 31-year-old man is placed on second-line triple therapy after a repeat endoscopy following an initial course has failed to eradicate *Helicobacter pylori* infection and ulceration. After the second course he returns to see his GP complaining of having a blackened tongue, nausea and dark stools.

14. THEME: MALABSORPTION

A Abetalipoproteinaemia
B Bacterial overgrowth
C Chronic pancreatitis
D Coeliac disease
E Crohn's disease
F Cystic fibrosis
G Giardiasis
H Short bowel syndrome
I Tuberculous terminal ileitis
J Tropical sprue

The following patients have all presented with malabsorption. Please choose the most appropriate diagnosis from the above list. Each diagnosis may be used once, more than once or not at all.

1. A 31-year-old Vietnamese man is referred to the Gastroenterology Out-patient's Clinic with a 2-month history of weight loss and loose, offensive stools. Initial investigations reveal a macrocytic anaemia and hypoalbuminaemia. The U&Es, LFTs, random blood glucose and thyroid function tests are all normal. His chest radiograph shows apical calcification and hilar lymphadenopathy. An upper endoscopy and small-bowel biopsy are unremarkable.

2. A 24-year-old woman is referred to the Gastroenterology Out-patients' Clinic with a 3-month history of weight loss, mouth ulceration, loose stools and lethargy. Initial investigations show: haemoglobin 10.4 g/dl, MCV 102 fl, WCC 9.2 × 10^9/l, platelets 399 × 10^9/l; Na$^+$ 132 mmol/l, K$^+$ 4.1 mmol/l, urea 4.1 mmol/l, creatinine 76 μmol/l; random blood glucose 4.9 mmol/l; total bilirubin 12 μmol/l, ALT 23 IU/l, AST 31 IU/l, alkaline phosphatase 56 IU/l, albumin 32 g/l; TSH 1.07 mU/1, fT4 23 pmol/l; anti-endomysial and anti-tissue glutaminase antibodies both highly positive.

3. A 49 year old man with a previous history of a Polya gastrectomy for gastric ulceration presents to his GP with a 3-month history of abdominal bloating, nausea, weight loss and steatorrhoea-like stools. He is referred to the local gastroenterologist and the diagnosis is subsequently confirmed by a positive ^{14}C breath test. He improves with a course of oral clarithromycin.

4. An 18 year old student returns from a 4-month trip around South-East Asia with a 6-week history of weight loss, diarrhoea, lethargy and malaise. On examination, he has obvious weight loss and is clinically anaemic. Abdominal examination is unremarkable. Stool microscopy and culture are negative for organisms, parasites, ova and cysts. A small-bowel biopsy confirms 'early villous stunting with increased crypt depth. No organisms are seen or cultured'. He improves with a course of folate, vitamin B$_{12}$ and tetracycline.

5. A 41-year-old chronic alcohol abuser presents to his GP with abdominal pain, lethargy and malaise associated with steatorrhoea-like stools. Initial investigations show: haemoglobin 9.1 g/dl, MCV 107 fl, WCC 4.2 × 10⁹/l, platelets 79 × 10⁹/l; Na⁺ 129 mmol/l, K⁺ 4.1 mmol/l, urea 3.1 mmol/l, creatinine 88 μmol/l; random blood glucose 12.9 mmol/l; total bilirubin 32 μmol/l, ALT 323 IU/l, AST 231 IU/l, alkaline phosphatase 356 IU/l, albumin 27 g/l; corrected Ca²⁺ 1.98 mmol/l, PO₄³⁻ 0.34 mmol/l. An abdominal radiograph shows 'speckled calcification across the upper abdomen'.

15. THEME: INFECTIVE DIARRHOEA

A   *Bacillus cereus*
B   *Campylobacter jejuni*
C   *Clostridium difficile*
D   *Cryptosporidium*
E   *Entamoeba histolytica*
F   *Giardia lamblia*
G   *Salmonella enteritidis*
H   *Salmonella typhi*
I   *Shigella*
J   *Vibrio cholerae*

The patients below have presented with infective diarrhoea. Please choose the most appropriate cause from the above list. Each option may be used once, more than once or not at all.

1. A 93-year-old woman is admitted to hospital with a severe chest infection. She requires 10 days of broad-spectrum antibiotics, nebulisers and oxygen before she improves. She is rehabilitating on the ward when she develops profuse, offensive, greenish diarrhoea.

2. A 22-year-old man is seen in the Emergency Department with severe abdominal cramps, vomiting and watery diarrhoea, several hours after eating the poorly reheated leftovers of last night's Chinese takeaway. Stool samples confirm Gram-positive, aerobic bacilli.

3. A middle-aged couple are seen by their GP at home with a 1-week history of severe, watery diarrhoea and 'foul-smelling belches', several days after returning from a trip to St Petersburg. Stool microscopy confirms the GP's initial diagnosis, showing cysts and trophozoites.

4. An aid worker returns from relief work in Bangladesh with a 3-day history of profuse, 'rice water'-like stools, vomiting and abdominal pains. Stool microscopy confirms the presence of a Gram-negative, rapidly motile bacillus whose movement in vitro is inhibited by type-specific antisera.

5. A 31-year-old, HIV-positive man is seen in the Emergency Department with profuse watery diarrhoea, weight loss and fever. His abdominal radiograph shows marked dilatation of his descending colon. Stool specimens confirm the presence of oocysts.

16. THEME: TYPES OF COLITIS

A Allergic colitis
B Amoebic colitis
C Collagenous colitis
D Crohn's colitis
E Diversion colitis
F Diverticular colitis
G Infective colitis
H Ischaemic colitis
I Lymphocytic colitis
J Pseudomembranous colitis
K Radiation colitis
L Ulcerative colitis

For each of the patients below, select the type of colitis that they are most likely to have from the above list. Each type may be used once, more than once or not at all.

1. A 21-year-old male student presents with a 2-month history of bloody diarrhoea with up to four stools per day. Colonoscopy shows diffuse mucosal erythema in continuity from the rectum to the mid-transverse colon. Repeat stool cultures are negative. Colonic biopsies show severe chronic inflammation limited to the mucosa, with crypt abscesses and crypt architectural distortion. L

2. A 75-year-old man who had an abdominal aortic aneurysm repair 10 days ago develops diarrhoea on the surgical ward. Colonoscopy shows ulceration at the splenic flexure. Repeat stool cultures are negative. K

3. A 12-year-old boy is brought to Paediatric Out-patients by his mother with a 9-month history of weight loss, abdominal pain and diarrhoea. On examination, he is on the 10th centile for height and weight, having been on the 50th centile at age of 10 years. Colonoscopy shows linear ulceration in the rectum, transverse colon and caecum, with normal mucosa in-between. Colonic biopsies show non-necrotising granulomas. D

4. A 45-year-old man receiving chemotherapy for lymphoma is treated with antibiotics for a chest infection brought on by neutropenia. Four days after starting antibiotics he develops profuse diarrhoea. Stool culture grows *Clostridium difficile*. J

5. A 53-year-old woman presents with a 3-month history of watery diarrhoea up to seven times per day. Colonoscopy is normal. Colonic biopsies show inflamed mucosa with a thickened subepithelial collagen band. C

6. A 35-year-old man presents with a 2-week history of profuse bloody diarrhoea and abdominal pain. Sigmoidoscopy in the Out-patients' Department reveals diffuse mucosal erythema in the rectum. Rectal biopsy shows oedema in the lamina propria and acute inflammation. Stool culture grows *Campylobacter jejuni*. G

17. THEME: INFLAMMATORY BOWEL DISEASE

A   Anterior uveitis
B   Autoimmune hepatitis
C   Cirrhosis
D   Episcleritis
E   Erythema nodosum
F   Gallstones
G   Oxalate renal stones
H   Pyoderma gangrenosum
I   Sacroiliitis
J   Sclerosing cholangitis

The following patients have all presented with extraintestinal manifestations of their inflammatory bowel disease. Please choose the most appropriate diagnosis from the above list. Each diagnosis may be used once, more than once or not at all..

1. A 34-year-old woman with known ulcerative colitis presents to her GP with a 2-week history of worsening jaundice. She is admitted to hospital where initial investigations reveal: haemoglobin 12.3 g/dl, MCV 86 fl, WCC 11.9 × 10⁹/l, platelets 209 × 10⁹/l; Na⁺ 137 mmol/l, K⁺ 4.8 mmol/l, urea 5.1 mmol/l, creatinine 87 µmol/l; total bilirubin 43 µmol/l, AST 378 IU/l, ALT 389 IU/l, alkaline phosphatase 643 IU/l, albumin 41 g/l. The diagnosis is subsequently confirmed by endoscopic retrograde cholangiopancreatography (ERCP), which shows 'beading' of the intrahepatic ducts.

     F x J

2. A 27-year-old man with long-standing Crohn's disease who has had several small-bowel resections presents in the Emergency Department with severe, right-sided loin pain, haematuria and rigors. Urine microscopy shows pus cells and red cells but no organisms.

    G

3. A 26-year-old man presents in the Emergency Department with a 6-week history of weight loss and the passage of blood and mucus per rectum associated with diarrhoea. He also complains of 'red, watery eyes', blurring of his vision and mild photophobia. A diagnosis of ulcerative colitis is confirmed on colonoscopy and biopsy.

    D x A

4. A 19-year-old woman presents in the Emergency Department with a 4-week history of abdominal pain and bloody diarrhoea. She has also noticed an enlarging 'ulcer' on her left shin.

    F x H

5. A 41-year-old man with known Crohn's disease presents in the Emergency Department with acute jaundice, nausea and vomiting and upper abdominal pain. On examination he is overtly icteric but not encephalopathic. There are no signs of chronic liver disease but he is pyrexial. Abdominal examination confirms a positive Murphy's sign. Subsequent blood cultures grow Gram-negative rods and an ERCP shows dilated bile ducts with a filling defect in the common bile duct.

    J x F

18. THEME: RECTAL BLEEDING

A   Anal carcinoma
B   Anal fissure
C   Colonic carcinoma
D   Colonic polyp
E   Crohn's disease
F   Diverticular disease
G   Haemorrhoids
H   Infective colitis
I   Ischaemic colitis
J   Ulcerative colitis

The patients below have all presented with rectal bleeding. Please select the most appropriate diagnosis from the above list. Each diagnosis may be used once, more than once or not at all.

1. A 64-year-old man presents with a 1-day history of dark-red rectal bleeding. He has complained of some diarrhoea for the last 6 months, and has noticed some loss of weight. Rectal examination and proctoscopy are normal. The FBC shows: haemoglobin 9.9 g/dl, MCV 84.3 fl, WCC 6.2 × 10⁹/l.

2. A 24-year-old woman presents with a 3-month history of lower abdominal colicky pain, diarrhoea (bowels opening six to ten times per day) and the passage of blood mixed with the stool. The FBC shows: haemoglobin 8.8 g/dl, MCV 78.6 fl, WCC 12.1 × 10⁹/l, ESR 62 mm/h.

3. A 54-year-old man with no previous abdominal symptoms complains of several episodes of painless, bright-red rectal bleeding, which is separate from the stool. Abdominal examination, rectal examination and proctoscopy are all normal. The FBC shows: haemoglobin 12.5 g/dl, WCC 5.4 × 10⁹/l.

4. A 24-year-old man presents with a 3-month history of episodes of painless, bright-red rectal bleeding on straining at stool. He has noticed some blood in the bowl, separate from the stool, and some on the paper after wiping. His haemoglobin is 13.7 g/dl.

5. A 28-year-old female medical student returns from her elective in Africa with a short history of severe lower abdominal cramps and the passage of bloody diarrhoea. Investigations show: haemoglobin 13.7 g/dl, WCC 13.2 × 10⁹/l; ESR 50 mm/h.

19. THEME: ANORECTAL CONDITIONS

A Anal carcinoma
B Anal fissure
C Anal fistula
D Anal skin tags
E Anal warts
F Haemorrhoids
G Perianal abscess
H Perianal haematoma
I Proctalgia fugax
J Rectal prolapse

The patients below have all presented with problems of the anorectum. Please select the most appropriate diagnosis from the above list. Each condition may be used once, more than once or not at all.

1. A 46-year-old man presents with a 3-month history of feeling a lump descending from the anal canal on defecation that he replaces into the anal canal digitally. He also gives a long history of bright-red bleeding per rectum, which is separate from the stool and noticeable on the paper.

2. A 70-year-old woman presents with a 6-month history of streaking of her stool with bright-red blood, anal pain and discharge. Examination reveals a raised, irregular ulcer on the anal verge.

3. An 80-year-old woman presents with a 6-month history of a large lump at the anus that appears after straining at stool and occasionally on standing and walking. She has also passed blood and mucus per rectum, and has faecal incontinence.

4. A 16-year-old boy complains of a 2-month history of pruritus ani, which he attributes to a watery, sometimes purulent discharge from the anus. On direct questioning, he has a 2 year history of right iliac fossa pain with occasional nausea and vomiting. He thinks that he might have lost a stone of so in weight over this time. Examination reveals some puckered scarring 2 cm from the anal verge, from which a small amount of pus can be expressed.

5. A 30-year-old man complains of a 2-day history of increasing anal pain that is made worse by sitting, moving or defecation. He has localised the source of the pain to a small lump on the verge of the anal canal. On examination, a deep-red/purple, hemispherical, 1-cm, hard lump is palpable at the anal margin.

20. THEME: COMMON ABDOMINAL OPERATIONS

A   Abdominoperineal excision of the rectum (APER)
B   Anterior resection of the rectum
C   Appendectomy
D   Emergency laparotomy
E   Hartmann's procedure
F   Left hemicolectomy
G   Oesophagectomy
H   Open cholecystectomy
I   Proctocolectomy with pouch ileoanal anastomosis (restorative proctocolectomy)
J   Right hemicolectomy

The patients below are all final MB examination long cases. Please select the most likely operation performed from the above list. Each operation may be used once, more than once or not at all.

1. A 72-year-old man tells you that he was admitted as an emergency with an acute abdomen caused by perforated diverticular disease. On examination, he has a healed, lower midline, vertical incision and a stoma sited in the left lower quadrant. The stoma is flush with the skin and the bag contains formed faeces.

2. A 23-year-old man with long-standing Crohn's disease gives you a long history from adolescence of recurrent episodes of small-intestinal obstruction caused by his disorder. He tells you that a 'special X-ray' demonstrated some narrowing of the bowel and that he has had the affected area of bowel removed. He is no longer symptomatic. Examination of the abdomen reveals a healed, vertical, midline incision.

3. A 48-year-old man with a prosthetic heart valve tells you that his abdominal problems started after a gunshot wound to the abdomen. He required a massive blood transfusion, had emergency surgery and spent some time in an intensive care unit. He has a long, vertical, midline surgical wound which now has a large incisional hernia.

4. A 40-year-old woman has long-standing ulcerative colitis. She tells you that she has had two operations. The first operation removed all of the affected bowel and left her with a 'bag' on the right side of the abdomen for some months. The second operation was to 'get rid of the bag'. She now suffers from some diarrhoea and urgency.

5. A 75-year-old woman gives a history of several months of rectal bleeding and passage of mucus before a cancer in the lower bowel was diagnosed. She had a 'major operation' 5 years ago. On examination, she has a lower vertical midline scar, a stoma on the left side (the bag contains formed faeces) and no anal opening.

21. THEME: ANATOMY OF THE INGUINAL REGION

A   Deep inguinal ring
B   Direct inguinal hernia
C   External oblique
D   Femoral hernia
E   Indirect inguinal hernia
F   Internal oblique
G   Mid-inguinal point
H   Mid-point of the inguinal ligament
I   Superficial inguinal ring
J   Transversalis fascia

The statements below are decribing hernias or anatomical features of the inguinal region. Please select the most appropriate hernia or anatomical description from the above list. Each option may be used once, more than once or not at all.

1. A 23-year-old male carpenter presents with a lump in the groin. Clinically, the lump lies above and medial to the pubic tubercle. At operation, the peritoneal sac is seen to arise at a point lateral to the inferior epigastric vessels.

2. At the operation for a groin lump in a 75-year-old man, a hernial sac lies between the lacunar ligament (medially) and the femoral vein (laterally).

3. A point whose surface marking is a point midway between the pubic tubercle and the anterior superior iliac spine. The position of the deep inguinal ring.

4. The aponeurosis of this muscle is incised from the point where the fibres divide medially to form the oval defect called the 'superficial inguinal ring', thus revealing the underlying inguinal canal and its contents.

5. As the spermatic cord passes through the inguinal canal it receives a covering from each of the three layers through which it passes. This layer forms the internal spermatic fascia.

22. THEME: HERNIAS

A   Incarcerated hernia
B   Incisional hernia
C   Lumbar hernia
D   Obstructed hernia
E   Obturator hernia
F   Richter's hernia
G   Sliding hernia
H   Spigelian hernia
I   Strangulated hernia
J   Umbilical hernia

The patients below all have hernias. Please select the most appropriate diagnosis from the above list. Each type of hernia may be used once, more than once or not at all.

1. A 53-year-old woman presents with a 2-day history of increasing colicky, central abdominal pain, nausea, vomiting and abdominal distension. On arrival in the Emergency Department she is in constant discomfort, febrile, very dehydrated and tachycardic. On abdominal examination, there is a large ventral hernia, which is irreducible and tender, with guarding and rebound. The overlying skin is red and oedematous.

2. A 33-year-old man complains of a painful lump along the lateral edge of the rectus sheath which is aggravated by strain and coughing. At operation, a hernia is found to be protruding through the semilunar line, which is formed by the aponeurosis of the internal oblique muscle at its point of division to enclose the rectus muscle.

3. A 46-year-old man presents with a left inguinoscrotal hernia. At operation by the ST3 doctor, a large indirect sac is noted. On incising the sac to reduce the contents, he is shocked to discover that he has made a cut into the lumen of the bowel, which is now leaking faeces.

4. A 53-year-old woman presents with a small swelling, immediately adjacent to and superior to her umbilicus. The swelling is irreducible but is not tender, and she has no gastrointestinal symptoms.

5. A 69-year-old man presents with a 2-day history of colicky central abdominal pain, vomiting and abdominal distension. On examination, he is noted to have a very large, irreducible but non-tender inguinoscrotal hernia.

23. THEME: ANATOMY OF THE LIVER

A   Caudate lobe
B   Caudate process
C   Coronary ligament
D   Falciform ligament
E   Left lobe
F   Left triangular ligament
G   Porta hepatis
H   Quadrate lobe
I   Right lobe
J   Right triangular ligament

For each of the statements below, choose the most appropriate structure from the above list. Each structure may be used once, more than once or not at all.

1. Lies medial to the body of the gallbladder. □

2. Is the site of entry of the portal vein into the liver. □

3. Encloses the bare area of the liver. □

4. Is related posteriorly to the oesophagus. □

5. Is a superior relation of the opening into the lesser sac. □

24. THEME: JAUNDICE

A   Autoimmune hepatitis
B   Budd–Chiari syndrome
C   Carcinoma of the head of pancreas
D   Cholangiocarcinoma
E   Gallstones
F   Gilbert's syndrome
G   Hepatitis A infection
H   Hepatitis B infection
I   Metastatic carcinoma
J   Primary biliary cirrhosis

The following patients have all presented with jaundice. Please choose the most appropriate diagnosis from the above list. Each diagnosis may be used once, more than once or not at all.

1. A 74-year-old man is seen in the Emergerncy Department with an acute chest infection. On examination, he is unwell, pyrexial and has icteric sclerae, with signs of right lower lobe pneumonia. His routine investigations reveal: haemoglobin 13.9 g/dl, MCV 81 fl, WCC 23.2 × 10⁹/l, platelets 307 × 10⁹/l; Na⁺ 141 mmol/l, K⁺ 4.6 mmol/l, urea 4.1 mmol/l, creatinine 71 μmol/l; random blood glucose 4.9 mmol/l; total bilirubin 37 μmol/l, AST 18 IU/l, ALT 19 IU/l, alkaline phosphatase 43 IU/l, albumin 41 g/l.

2. A 41-year-old man is seen in the Emergemcy Department with acute jaundice, nausea and vomiting and diarrhoea, 3 weeks after returning from South-East Asia. Initial investigations show: total bilirubin 43 μmol/l, AST 432 IU/l, ALT 522 IU/l, alkaline phosphatase 177 IU/l, albumin 35 g/l; INR 1.2. An acute-phase IgM response is demonstrated.

3. A 61-year-old woman with known polycythaemia rubra vera is admitted to hospital with worsening jaundice and pruritus. On examination, she is icteric and she has tender hepatomegaly, ascites, and peripheral oedema, including a marked sacral pad. The diagnosis is demonstrated by ultrasound scan of the abdomen and a venogram of the inferior vena cava and hepatic vein.

4. A 52-year-old woman is seen in the Gastroenterology Out-patient Clinic with a 6-week history of worsening jaundice, pruritus and weight loss. On examination, she has spider naevi, hepatomegaly and jaundice. Investigations show: antimitochondrial antibodies strongly positive; anti-smooth muscle antibodies and anti-LKM (liver, kidney, microsomal) antibodies both negative.

5. An obese 71-year-old man is referred to Surgical Out-patients with a 2-week history of worsening jaundice associated with dark urine and pale stools. An ultrasound scan arranged by the GP is reported as: 'a technically difficult study showing a dilated common bile duct and gallbladder but no gallstones identified. The pancreas and spleen were poorly visualised – recommend ERCP'. The diagnosis is subsequently confirmed by ERCP and abdominal CT.

25. THEME: DISEASES OF THE LIVER

A Alcoholic hepatitis
B α_1-Antitrypsin deficiency
C Ascending cholangitis
D Budd–Chiari syndrome
E Chronic hepatitis B
F Genetic haemochromatosis
G Hepatitis C
H Primary biliary cirrhosis
I Primary sclerosing cholangitis
J Wilson's disease

For each of the patients below, select the most likely liver disease from the above list. Each diagnosis may be used once, more than once or not at all.

1. A 47-year-old woman presents with recent onset of jaundice. On further questioning, she has had bouts of pruritus for several months. Liver function tests are abnormal, with a moderately raised bilirubin, a very high alkaline phosphatase and normal transaminases. Other tests include a raised IgM and high serum cholesterol. An autoantibody screen shows antimitochondrial antibodies in a titre of 1 : 256. A liver biopsy shows expansion of the portal tracts by lymphocytes and plasma cells and occasional granulomas; bile ducts are scarce.

2. A 42-year-old African man presents to a preoperative assessment clinic prior to laparoscopic cholecystectomy. Routine liver function tests are abnormal with high transaminases but normal bilirubin and normal alkaline phosphatase. Further investigations include a liver biopsy, which shows moderate to severe chronic inflammation with moderate fibrosis. Special stains identify antigens from a double-stranded DNA virus within the cytoplasm of many hepatocytes.

3. A 51-year-old man presents to his GP complaining of pain in the right hypochondrium. On examination, there is hepatomegaly 2 cm below the costal margin. The GP also notices that the patient's skin appears to have darkened since his last visit to the surgery several years ago. Liver function tests ordered by the GP show markedly raised transaminases with a normal bilirubin and normal alkaline phosphatase. He is referred to the local hospital where a liver biopsy is carried out. This shows cirrhosis and heavy deposition of haemosiderin within the cytoplasm of hepatocytes and bile duct epithelium.

4. A 61-year-old woman with known polycythaemia rubra vera presents with a short history of nausea, vomiting and abdominal pain. On examination, she has tender hepatomegaly 3 cm below the costal margin and moderate ascites. Liver function tests show mildly elevated transaminases, bilirubin at the upper end of the normal range and a normal alkaline phosphatase. Liver biopsy shows features consistent with venous outflow obstruction.

5. A 17-year-old boy presents with symptoms and signs of chronic liver disease. Liver function tests show high transaminases with a normal bilirubin and normal alkaline phosphatase. Liver biopsy shows chronic inflammation in the portal tracts accompanied by moderate to severe fibrosis. There is prominent accumulation of copper-associated protein in periportal hepatocytes. After the liver biopsy the serum caeruloplasmin and copper levels are measured – both are lower than normal.

26. THEME: DRUG-INDUCED JAUNDICE

A Amiodarone
B Azathioprine
C Carbamazepine
D Chlorpromazine
E Erythromycin
F Haloperidol
G Lisinopril
H Nifedipine
I Phenytoin
J Rifampicin

The following patients have all presented with jaundice secondary to their medication. Please choose the most likely responsible agent from the above list. Each drug may be used once, more than once or not at all.

1. A 31-year-old man is admitted to hospital with a diagnosis of possible *Legionella* pneumonia. Investigations confirm hyponatraemia and mildly deranged LFTs. His chest radiograph shows hazy shadowing in the left mid- and lower zones. He is started on an antibiotic but 5 days later he becomes acutely jaundiced with red discoloration of his urine and tears.

2. A 19-year-old woman is seen by her GP because she has a severe sore throat, for which he prescribes an antibiotic. Five days later she returns with a yellowish discoloration of her sclera. Her LFTs show: total bilirubin 36 μmol/l, AST 56 IU/l, ALT 62 IU/l, alkaline phoshpatase 167 IU/l, albumin 41 g/l.

3. A previously fit and well, 81-year-old man is admitted to hospital with a collapse. A 24-hour ECG tape shows episodes of atrial fibrillation with a rate between 130 bpm and 170 bpm. He is started on treatment and is discharged. Six weeks later he returns to the Out-patients' Department and is noted to be jaundiced. His admission LFTs had been normal.

4. A 51-year-old woman with type 2 diabetes is started on treatment for hypertension by her GP. Several weeks later she returns to see the GP regarding a dry, irritating cough. She is reassured that it might be due to the medication and that if it continues she might have to stop the tablets. A week later she returns with jaundice. Her LFTs show: total bilirubin 39 μmol/l, AST 57 IU/l, ALT 53 IU/l, alkaline phosphatase 277 IU/l, albumin 37 g/l. The medication is withdrawn on the advice of the local gastroenterologist and her symptoms improve. Subsequent LFTs are normal.

5. A 41-year-old man with known rheumatoid arthritis is started on a new treatment in Rheumatology Outpatients. He is not feeling well and cancels his next appointment but is then seen in the Emergency Department with acute jaundice. The LFTs show: total bilirubin 41 μmol/l, AST 47 IU/l, ALT 51 IU/l, alkaline phosphatase 211 IU/l, albumin 40 g/l. An ultrasound scan of the abdomen is unremarkable. The LFTs return to normal on stopping the new medication.

27. THEME: ASCITES

A   Abdominal trauma
B   Acute pancreatitis
C   Alcoholic cirrhosis
D   Bacterial peritonitis
E   Congestive cardiac failure
F   Hepatic vein occlusion
G   Malignant mesothelioma
H   Nephrotic syndrome
I   Ovarian carcinoma
J   Tuberculosis

For each of the descriptions below, select the condition that is most likely to be causing the associated ascites from the above list. Each option may be used once, more than once or not at all.

1. Adenocarcinoma cells in the ascitic fluid. ☐

2. Granulomas in the ascitic fluid. ☐

3. Hypercholesterolaemia. ☐

4. A very high serum amylase concentration. ☐

5. A very high serum concentration of γ-glutamyltransferase. ☐

28. THEME: DISORDERS OF THE PANCREAS

A Acute haemorrhagic pancreatitis
B Adenocarcinoma
C Annular pancreas
D Chronic pancreatitis
E Cystadenoma
F Gastrinoma
G Heterotopic pancreas
H Insulinoma
I Pancreas divisum
J Pancreatic pseudocyst

For each of the patients below, select the most likely pancreatic disorder from the above list. Each disorder may be used once, more than once or not at all.

1. A 45-year-old man presents with a 6-month history of epigastric pain that has recently worsened. The pain is worse at night and is relieved by antacids. Endoscopy shows gastric mucosal erythema and several peptic ulcers distributed throughout the first, second and third parts of the duodenum.

2. A 36-year-old woman with a long history of gallstones presents to the Emergency Department with a 12-hour history of severe abdominal pain radiating to the back. On examination, she is tachycardic, tachypnoeic and hypotensive. Investigations show a mildly raised bilirubin and a serum amylase level that is six times above normal. An abdominal ultrasound shows a stone in the common bile duct.

3. A 75-year-old woman presents with a 1-week history of painless obstructive jaundice. A CT scan shows a 5-cm mass in the head of the pancreas. Fine-needle aspiration of this mass shows malignant glandular cells.

4. A 56-year-old man, a known chronic alcoholic, presents with repeated attacks of abdominal pain precipitated by bouts of heavy drinking. The pain radiates to his back and is relieved by leaning forwards. On further questioning he admits to having loose, pale, greasy stools that are difficult to flush. A plain abdominal radiograph reveals calcification in the peritoneal cavity.

5. A 20-year-old male university student is brought into the Emergency Department having fainted during a rugby match. On questioning he says he felt dizzy for several minutes, developed palpitations and then suddenly blacked out. He admits that he has suffered similar episodes in the past, always related to sport or exercise.

CHAPTER **2**

Genitourinary

1. THEME: ANATOMY OF THE GENITOURINARY SYSTEM

A Body of the uterus
B Ejaculatory duct
C Membranous urethra
D Ovary
E Penile urethra
F Prostatic urethra
G Seminal vesicle
H Trigone of the bladder
I Uterine tube
J Vas deferens

For each of the statements below choose the most appropriate structure from the above list. Each structure may be used once, more than once or not at all.

1. Develops from the fused caudal ends of the mesonephric ducts. ☐

2. Formed by the caudal fusion of the paramesonephric (Müllerian) ducts. ☐

3. Overlies the origin of the internal iliac artery. ☐

4. Lies between the neck of the bladder and the fascia of the pelvic floor. ☐

5. Lies within the deep perineal pouch. ☐

2. THEME: URINARY TRACT AND RELATED ANATOMY

A   Female pelvic ureter
B   Left abdominal ureter
C   Left kidney
D   Left renal pelvis
E   Left adrenal gland
F   Male pelvic ureter
G   Right abdominal ureter
H   Right kidney
I   Right renal pelvis
J   Right adrenal gland

For each of the statements below, choose the most appropriate structure from the above list. Each structure may be used once, more than once or not at all.

1. Crossed by the ileocolic artery.

2. Crossed by the left uterine artery.

3. Related to the bare area of the liver.

4. Covered anteriorly by the curve of the duodenum.

5. Related to the distal end of the transverse colon.

3. THEME: HAEMATURIA I

A Anticoagulant therapy
B Bladder cancer
C Catheter trauma
D Cystitis
E Glomerulonephritis
F Haemophilia
G Polycystic kidney disease
H Prostate cancer
I Renal-cell carcinoma
J Ureteric calculus

The patients below have all presented with blood in the urine. Please select the most appropriate diagnosis from the above list. Each diagnosis may be used once, more than once or not at all.

1. An 86-year-old man presents with a 3-day history of noticing frank blood in his urine, especially at the start of the stream. He has recently been investigated for urinary frequency and hesitancy, but failed to attend his out-patient investigations. On direct questioning, he also notes some lower back pain for several months. Investigations show: haemoglobin 9.7 g/dl, WCC 10.2 × 10⁹/l; urea 11.1 mmol/l, creatinine 92 μmol/l; prostate-specific antigen (PSA) 644 nmol/l. H ☐

2. A 78-year-old man presents with a 12-hour history of passing heavily bloodstained urine. He is a smoker and worked in the rubber industry in the 1950s. He has no other symptoms and examination is unremarkable. Investigations show: haemoglobin 11.2 g/dl, WCC 8.6 × 10⁹/l; urea 4.5 mmol/l, creatinine 98 μmol/l; PSA 8 nmol/l. B ☐

3. A 40-year-old man presents with macroscopic haematuria throughout the urine stream. Abdominal examination reveals bilateral ballotable masses in the flanks. Investigations show: haemoglobin 13.2 g/dl, WCC 6.0 × 10⁹/l; urea 22.3 mmol/l, creatinine 345 μmol/l; PSA 2 nmol/l. G ☐

4. For 2 months a 60-year-old man has noticed some blood in his urine, mixed throughout the stream. He also has some right loin pain. Examination reveals a right loin mass. Investigations show: haemoglobin 9.9 g/dl, WCC 8.2 × 10⁹/l; urea 10.1 mmol/l, creatinine 112 μmol/l; ESR 80 mm/h. I ☐

5. A 34-year-old man presents with a 4-hour history of sudden-onset, severe left loin pain, radiating to the groin. Examination is unremarkable. Urinalysis demonstrates microscopic haematuria. Investigations show: haemoglobin 14.8 g/dl, WCC 9.2 × 10⁹/l; urea 6.1 mmol/l, creatinine 68 μmol/l. J ☐

4. THEME: HAEMATURIA II

A   Bladder calculi
B   *Escherichia coli* infection
C   Glomerulonephritis
D   Polycystic kidneys
E   Pyelonephritis
F   Renal calculi
G   Renal-cell carcinoma
H   Renal tuberculosis
I   Staphylococcal infection
J   Transitional-cell carcinoma of the bladder

The patients below have presented with frank haematuria. Please choose the most appropriate diagnosis from the above list. Each diagnosis may be used once, more than once or not at all.

1. A 17-year-old girl presents to the Emergency Department with a 3-month history of worsening dull loin pain and haematuria. On examination, she is plethoric and hypertensive, with a BP of 195/110 mmHg. Examination of her abdomen reveals bilateral ballotable masses in the lumbar regions. Of note, her grandmother died suddenly of a brain haemorrhage at the age of 34.

2. A 41-year-old woman with known renal stones presents to her GP with a 3-day history of nausea and vomiting, right-sided loin pain and rigors. On examination, she is pyrexial and tachycardic, her BP is 110/70 mmHg and abdominal examination reveals severe tenderness in the right loin. Urinalysis shows: blood ++, protein ++, nitrites ++.

3. A 54-year-old Pakistani man presents to his GP with a 3-month history of weight loss and night sweats. He is admitted to hospital for further investigations. Examination is unremarkable other than some axillary and inguinal lymphadenopathy and obvious weight loss. His observation chart shows a low-grade pyrexia with occasional spikes to 38.5 °C. Initial midstream urine (MSU) and urine cytology is negative but an early-morning urine (EMU) shows the presence of acid and alcohol-fast bacilli (AAFB).

4. A 37-year-old man presents to Medical Out-patients with a 6-month history of recurrent left-sided abdominal pain. An MSU sample sent by the GP shows a WCC of >1000/mm³, no organisms or casts seen. A plain abdominal radiograph is unremarkable but an intravenous pyelogram (IVP) shows an obstructed left pelvicalyceal system with a filling defect in the proximal left ureter.

5. An 87-year-old woman presents in the Emergency Department with increasing confusion and falls. On examination, she is apyrexial but is flushed and is very confused, with an abridged mental test score (AMTS) of 3/10. Clinically, she is in fast atrial fibrillation and has a BP of 100/60 mmHg, but otherwise respiratory, cardiovascular, abdominal and neurological examinations are unremarkable. Subsequent MSU shows 'Gram-negative rods sensitive to trimethoprim and amoxicillin'.

5. THEME: HYPOALBUMINAEMIA

A   Carcinomatosis
B   Chronic renal failure
C   Cirrhosis
D   Malabsorption
E   Malnutrition
F   Nephrotic syndrome
G   Pregnancy
H   Protein-losing enteropathy
I   Septicaemia
J   Severe burns

The patients below have all presented with hypoalbuminaemia. Please choose the most appropriate diagnosis from the above list. Each diagnosis may be used once, more than once or not at all.

1. A previously fit and well, 81-year-old man is admitted to hospital with a 5-day history of confusion and abdominal pain. Examination in the Emergency Department reveals a BP of 90/60 mmHg, pulse 120 bpm irregular, but little else of note. Investigations show: WCC 21.3 × 10⁹/l; Na⁺ 159 mmol/l, K⁺ 5.4 mmol/l, urea 18 mmol/l, creatinine 120 µmol/l. Urinalysis showed: blood ++, protein ++, nitrites +. He recovers with treatment but 6 days later his albumin, which was initially 39 g/l, has dropped to 27 g/l.

2. A 42-year-old woman presents to her GP with a 3-month history of worsening pruritus, jaundice and abdominal swelling. Subsequent investigations reveal: total bilirubin 132 µmol/l, aspartate transaminase (AST) 1023 IU/l, alanine transaminase (ALT) 904 IU/l, alkaline phosphatase 657 IU/l; international normalised ratio (INR) 2.1; anti-smooth muscle and antimitochondrial antibodies strongly positive.

3. A 22-year-old woman presents to her GP with a 6-month history of severe malaise, lethargy, diarrhoea and weight loss. Investigations reveal: haemoglobin 9.1 g/dl, mean corpuscular volume (MCV) 102 fl, WCC 4.7 × 10⁹/l, platelets 143 × 10⁹/l; urea and electrolytes (U&Es) normal; albumin 25 g/l, liver function tests (LFTs) otherwise normal; red cell folate 1.2 mg/l; antiendomysial antibody strongly positive.

4. A 48-year-old man is referred to the Gastroenterology Clinic with a 1-year history of weight loss, diarrhoea, arthralgia and recent ankle oedema. Investigations reveal: hamoglobin 8.4 g/dl, MCV 86 fl, WCC 8.2 × 10⁹/l (eosinophilia noted), platelets 651 × 10⁹/l; albumin 21 g/l, LFTs otherwise normal. Subsequent small-bowel biopsy reveals 'stunted villi with PAS-positive macrophages and Gram-positive bacilli' (PAS = periodic acid–Schiff [stain]).

5. A 19-year-old female medical student presents to her local GP with malaise. She is accompanied by her flatmate, who is concerned about her gross weight loss and 'fanatical' exercise programme over the last term. Her body mass index (BMI) is 16 kg/m².

6. THEME: GLOMERULONEPHRITIS

A   Anti-glomerular basement membrane disease
B   Bronchial carcinoma
C   Diabetes mellitus
D   Henoch–Schönlein purpura
E   Hepatitis B
F   Hodgkin's lymphoma
G   Infective endocarditis
H   Sickle-cell disease
I   Streptococcal pneumonia
J   Systemic lupus erythematosus

The patients below have all presented with glomerulonephritis. Please choose the most appropriate diagnosis from the above list. Each diagnosis may be used once, more than once or not at all.

1. A 37-year-old man presents to his GP with increasing shortness of breath associated with a dry cough, haemoptysis and ankle oedema, several days after having a flu-like illness associated with pharyngitis. Investigations reveal: Na$^+$ 131 mmol/l, K$^+$ 5.8 mmol/l, urea 23.3 mmol/l, and creatinine 453 μmol/l, A chest radiograph shows patchy shadowing throughout the lung fields.

2. A previously fit and well, 87-year-old woman presents to the Emergency Department with a 2-month history of malaise associated with increasing shortness of breath and ankle oedema. On examination, she is pyrexial, has tender nodules in the pulps of her fingers and a harsh systolic murmur is heard throughout the praecordium.

3. A 12-year-old schoolboy presents with a spreading rash over his shins, associated with abdominal pain, malaise and ankle oedema. His anti-streptolysin-O titre (ASOT) is negative and blood cultures are negative.

4. A 34-year-old man presents to the Emergency Department with a 2-month history of malaise, lethargy, night sweats and ankle and finger swelling. On examination, he is apyrexial but has axillary, cervical and submandibular lymphadenopathy associated with hepatosplenomegaly. His chest radiograph shows bilateral hilar lymphadenopathy.

5. A 54-year-old smoker presents to his GP with a 2-month history of increasing exertional dyspnoea, ankle oedema and several episodes of haemoptysis. On examination, he is apyrexial but has cervical lymphadenopathy and is cachectic. Chest examination reveals coarse crackles and bronchial breathing at the right base.

7. THEME: CHRONIC INTERSTITIAL NEPHRITIS

A   Alport's syndrome
B   Balkan nephropathy
C   Chronic pyelonephritis
D   Diabetes mellitus
E   Heavy metal toxicity
F   Hyperuricaemic nephropathy
G   NSAIDs
H   Radiotherapy
I   Sickle-cell disease
J   Sjögren's syndrome

The patients below have all presented with chronic interstitial nephritis. Please choose the most appropriate diagnosis from the above list. Each diagnosis may be used once, more than once or not at all.

1. A 61-year-old woman with chronic back pain presents to the Emergency Department with a 3-month history of worsening dyspeptic pain and a single episode of frank haematemesis. Investigations reveal: haemoglobin 8.5 g/dl, MCV 69 fl, WCC 11.5 × 10^9/l, platelets 543 × 10^9/l; Na$^+$ 129 mmol/l, K$^+$ 6.4 mmol/l, urea 28 mmol/l, creatinine 620 μmol/l.

2. A 17-year-old woman is referred to the Renal Out-patient Department with abnormal U&Es and a history of recurrent urinary tract infections. Investigations reveal: Na$^+$ 127 mmol/l, K$^+$ 6.8 mmol/l, urea 32 mmol/l, creatinine 620 μmol/l, corrected Ca^{2+} 1.98 mmol/l, and PO$_4^{3-}$ 2.09 mmol/l. An ultrasound scan of the renal tract shows bilaterally shrunken kidneys.

3. A 37-year-old Afro-Caribbean man presents to his GP with severe abdominal pain and headaches 3 days after developing a sore throat and dry cough. This is his third such admission in the last 5 months. Investigations reveal: haemoglobin 5.5 g/dl, MCV 81 fl, WCC 13.5 × 10^9/l, platelets 243 × 10^9/l; Na$^+$ 131 mmol/l, K$^+$ 4.9 mmol/l, urea 14.2 mmol/l, and creatinine 320 μmol/l. Urinalysis shows: blood +++, protein +++, nitrites negative.

4. A 50-year-old man with a history of ischaemic heart disease (IHD) and hyperlipidaemia presents to his GP with increasing lethargy and ankle oedema. Routine investigations reveal: haemoglobin 13.5 g/dl, MCV 86.8 fl, WCC 7.5 × 10^9/l, platelets 231 × 10^9/l; Na$^+$ 127 mmol/l, K$^+$ 5.3 mmol/l, urea 24.7 mmol/l, creatinine 500 μmol/l, glucose 23.1 mmol/l and haemoglobin A$_{1c}$ (Hb A$_{1c}$) 13.5%.

5. An 11-year-old deaf boy presents to his GP with haematuria, worsening lethargy and ankle oedema. Investigations reveal acute on chronic renal failure, with deranged U&Es, hypoalbuminaemia and hypocalcaemia.

8. THEME: NEPHROTIC SYNDROME

A Amyloidosis
B Anaphylaxis
C Diabetes mellitus
D Gold therapy
E IgA nephropathy
F Malaria
G Minimal-change nephropathy
H Penicillamine
I Polyarteritis nodosa
J Wegener's granulomatosis

The patients below have all presented with features of nephrotic syndrome. Please choose the most appropriate diagnosis from the above list. Each diagnosis may be used once, more than once or not at all.

1. A 39-year-old woman with long-standing rheumatoid arthritis presents to her GP with increasing swelling of the hands, face and legs, associated with being unable to taste her food, 6 weeks after starting a new treatment.

2. A 17-year-old student presents in the Emergency Department with a 6-day history of a sore throat and flu-like symptoms, now associated with frank haematuria, swelling of her ankles and poor urine output. She has had two episodes of pharyngitis in the last 3 weeks.

3. A 27-year-old man presents to his GP with nasal discharge, a dry cough associated with two episodes of haemoptysis and swollen legs. Subsequent investigations confirm a nephrotic syndrome associated with an extremely high cytoplasmic antineutrophil cytoplasmic antibody (c-ANCA) titre.

4. A 69-year-old man returns from Nigeria with increasing leg oedema and pyrexia. Investigations reveal a reticulocytosis, thrombocytopenia and intracellular 'inclusion bodies' in his red cells.

5. A 19-year-old student presents to his GP with a 2-week history of malaise and swelling of his hands and feet, associated with passing very small volumes of urine for the past 3 days. Subsequent renal biopsy confirms loss of the renal epithelial podocytes, with no other significant pathology identified.

9. THEME: CALCIFICATION OF THE RENAL TRACT

A Calcium oxalate stones
B Carcinoma of the bladder
C Hydatid cyst
D Hyperparathyroidism
E Medullary sponge kidney
F Prostatic calculi
G Renal carcinoma
H Schistosomiasis
I Staghorn calculus
J Tuberculosis

The patients below have all presented with disorders leading to calcification of their renal tract. Please choose the most appropriate cause from the above list. Each option may be used once, more than once or not at all.

1. A retired Welsh hill farmer presents to his GP with a 3-month history of vague right upper quadrant pain. Many years ago he had been admitted with 'cysts' in the liver and kidney but these were removed. A plain abdominal radiograph shows calcification on the right of L2/3 and in the right upper quadrant. His FBC, U&Es and LFTs are all normal.

2. A 63-year-old botanist presents to his GP with a 2-week history of suprapubic pain and frank haematuria associated with fever and weight loss. He has recently returned from a sabbatical in Africa. His MSU shows blood +++, protein +++, and nitrites negative, and an abdominal radiograph reveals calcification of the bladder.

3. A 49-year-old Bangladeshi man presents to his GP with non-specific abdominal pains and right-sided chest pain. A chest radiograph reveals apical calcification and an abdominal radiograph shows bilateral calcification at the level of the kidneys. His FBC, U&Es and LFTs are normal and his pain is eased with paracetamol.

4. A 41-year-old woman presents to her GP with a 'multitude of symptoms' including loin pains, constipation, lethargy and an inability to concentrate. Examination is unremarkable. Investigations reveal: Na^+ 136 mmol/l, K^+ 5.0 mmol/l, urea 4.1 mmol/l, creatinine 60 μmol/l, corrected Ca^{2+} 3.42 mmol/l, PO_4^{3-} 0.89 mmol/l; ESR 14 mm/h.

5. A 78-year-old woman presents to the Emergency Department with severe left-sided loin pain and rigors. On examination, she is in severe pain, pyrexial (40 °C) and has left-sided abdominal tenderness. Her abdominal radiograph shows a large, irregular, calcified mass in the left upper quadrant. Culture of her urine reveals a *Proteus* infection.

10. THEME: RENAL MASSES

A   Hydronephrosis
B   Nephroblastoma
C   Perinephric abscess
D   Polycystic kidney disease
E   Renal abscess
F   Renal amyloidosis
G   Renal-cell carcinoma
H   Renal cyst
I   Transplanted kidney

The patients below have all presented with a renal mass. Please choose the most likely diagnosis from the above list. Each diagnosis may be used once, more than once or not at all.

1. A 27-year-old woman presents to her GP with insidious worsening of lethargy, nausea and pruritus. She is plethoric, has a BP of 200/120 mmHg and has bilateral abdominal masses. She is referred to the medical team on call and routine blood tests reveal: haemoglobin 16.2 g/dl, haematocrit 0.54, WCC 9.2×10^9/l, platelets 197×10^9/l; Na$^+$127 mmol/l, K$^+$ 6.9 mmol/l, urea 67.5 mmol/l, creatinine 1020 μmol/l.

2. A 39-year-old man with long-standing rheumatoid arthritis presents in the Out-patients' Department with oliguria and peripheral oedema. Rectal biopsy confirms apple-green positive birefringence when stained with Congo red and viewed under polarised light.

3. A 5-year-old girl presents with an increasingly swollen abdomen and haematuria associated with malaise and fever. Ultrasound scan shows a large mass in the left kidney.

4. A 79-year-old man presents with a 6-month history of worsening prostatism associated with a 2-week history of oliguria and oedema. On examination he has a palpable bladder and kidneys. Investigations show: Na$^+$ 131 mmol/l, K$^+$ 6.2 mmol/l, urea 39 mmol/l, creatinine 506 μmol/l, PSA 97.6 nmol/l.

5. A thin 54-year-old man is admitted to hospital for a routine inguinal hernia repair. On examination, the ST4 doctor is able to ballot the right kidney and orders an ultrasound scan of the renal tract. The scan confirms a normal left kidney and a normal pelvicalyceal system on the right with a large fluid-filled area in the right upper pole, measuring 10 cm × 8 cm.

11. THEME: POLYCYSTIC KIDNEY DISEASE

A   Haematuria
B   Hepatosplenomegaly
C   Hypertension
D   Polycythaemia
E   Recurrent urinary tract infection
F   Renal calculi
G   Renal-cell carcinoma
H   Subarachnoid haemorrhage

The patients below have all presented with complications of adult polycystic kidney disease (APCKD). Please choose the most appropriate diagnosis from the above list. Each diagnosis may be used once, more than once or not at all.

1. A 27-year-old woman with known APCKD presents in the Emergency Department with sudden collapse. She had complained to her boss of a severe headache that morning and had been forced to go home because of its severity. On examination, she has a Glasgow Coma Scale (GCS) score of 3, BP 170/100 mmHg and pulse 40 bpm. Fundoscopy reveals papilloedema.

2. A 17-year-old girl with APCKD presents to her GP with a 1-week history of a mild dull headache. On examination, her BP is 185/105 mmHg, pulse 88 bpm and regular, and she has bilaterally palpable kidneys. Fundoscopy reveals normal discs but arteriovenous (AV) nipping and occasional exudates.

3. A 22-year-old man presents to his GP with a 2-month history of exertional dyspnoea and ankle oedema. On examination, he is plethoric, his cardiovascular and respiratory examinations are unremarkable, but he has a palpable mass in the left flank and possible hepatomegaly. He has pitting oedema of his ankles. Investigations show: haemoglobin 18.9 g/dl, haematocrit 0.57, MCV 87 fl, WCC 10.2×10^9/l, platelets 187×10^9/l; Na^+ 131 mmol/l, K^+ 6.2 mmol/l, urea 34.2 mmol/l, creatinine 1011 μmol/l.

4. A 34-year-old man with known APCKD presents with a 2-month history of night sweats, haematuria and dull loin pain. Urinalysis and MSU confirm the presence of large amounts of blood and protein in the urine but no pus or organisms are seen. An ultrasound scan shows a solid mass in the upper pole of the right kidney.

5. A 28-year-old woman with known APCKD presents to her GP with a 2-day history of rigors, vomiting and haematuria, associated with left loin pain and tenderness. On examination, she is unwell, temperature 38.5 °C, BP 95/60 mmHg, pulse 120 bpm and thready. Urinalysis shows blood +++, protein ++, nitrites ++. She is admitted to hospital where subsequent investigations confirm Gram-negative rods in her urine and blood cultures.

12. THEME: TUMOURS OF THE URINARY TRACT

A   Adenocarcinoma
B   Angiomyolipoma
C   Haemangioma
D   Nephroblastoma
E   Oncocytoma
F   Renal-cell carcinoma
G   Renal cortical adenoma
H   Renal fibroma
I   Squamous-cell carcinoma
J   Transitional-cell carcinoma

For each of the patients below, select the most likely urinary tract tumour from the above list. Each tumour may be used once, more than once or not at all.

1. A 55-year-old man presents with a 1-month history of left loin pain and a 2-day history of painless haematuria. On examination he has a palpable loin mass. A CT scan shows a poorly circumscribed, 10-cm tumour located in the upper pole of the left kidney. The tumour involves the left adrenal gland and extends into the left renal vein. Histology shows a clear-cell tumour.

2. A 67-year-old woman who worked in the textile-dying industry for many years presents with a 1-week history of painless haematuria. Culture of the urine is negative but cytology shows atypical transitional cells. Cystoscopy shows a 3-cm lesion with a papillary surface located at the trigone.

3. A 12-month-old boy presents to the paediatricians with abdominal distension. Investigations show a 6-cm mass in the right kidney. Histology of the excised mass shows a malignant 'embryonic' neoplasm.

4. A 42-year-old Egyptian man presents with haematuria. Culture of the urine is negative. Cystoscopy shows a large mass in the posterior wall of the bladder, and a biopsy of this shows a malignant tumour with foci of keratinisation. Clusters of schistosome ova are scattered throughout the biopsy.

5. A 22-year-old woman with known tuberose sclerosis is found to have a well-circumscribed, 8-cm mass in the lower pole of the right kidney. Histology of the excised mass shows a benign tumour composed of blood vessels, muscle and mature fat.

13. THEME: RENAL FAILURE

A   Benign prostatic hypertrophy
B   Carcinoma of the prostate
C   Diabetes mellitus
D   Diclofenac
E   Haemorrhage
F   Henoch–Schönlein purpura
G   IgA nephropathy
H   Multiple myeloma
I   Renal artery stenosis
J   Rhabdomyolysis

The patients below have all presented with renal failure. Please choose the most appropriate diagnosis from the above list. Each diagnosis may be used once, more than once or not at all.

1. A 35-year-old alcohol abuser presents to the Emergency Department with confusion and melaena. On examination, he has several signs of chronic liver disease and is pale and clammy. His BP is 90/50 mmHg and he has a weak thready pulse of 130 bpm. Investigations reveal: haemoglobin 6.3 g/dl, MCV 108 fl, WCC 3.8 × 10⁹/l, platelets 23 × 10⁹/l; Na⁺ 123 mmol/l, K⁺ 4.4 mmol/l, urea 27 mmol/l, creatinine 123 μmol/l.

2. A 74-year-old man presents to his GP with increasing malaise and back pain associated with hesitancy and poor urinary stream. Subsequent investigations reveal: Na⁺ 134 mmol/l, K⁺ 6.4 mmol/l, urea 31.2 mmol/l, creatinine 1023 μmol/l; and PSA 123 nmol/l. An ultrasound scan shows bilateral hydronephrotic kidneys.

3. A 61-year-old woman with known peripheral vascular disease and IHD is started on an angiotensin-converting enzyme (ACE) inhibitor by her GP. Three weeks later she is admitted to hospital with increasing confusion and pruritus. Investigations reveal: haemoglobin 12.3 g/dl, MCV 85.2 fl, WCC 6.8 × 10⁹/l, platelets 403 × 10⁹/l; Na⁺ 130 mol/l, K⁺ 7.4 mol/l, urea 37 mmol/l, and creatinine 841 μmol/l. Urinalysis shows: protein ++, ketones +, no blood.

4. An 84-year-old woman is found on the floor of her flat by a neighbour. She had had a fall 3 days prior to her 'rescue' and had been unable to get up or raise the alarm. On admission to hospital, investigations reveal: haemoglobin 15.3 g/dl, MCV 91.2 fl, WCC 23.1 × 10⁹/l, platelets 403 × 10⁹/l; Na⁺ 145 mmol/l, K⁺ 7.1 mmol/l, urea 32.9 mmol/l, creatinine 649 μmol/l, creatine kinase 23,089 IU/l.

5. A 24-year-old man presents to his GP with an increasing rash over his lower limbs and buttocks associated with arthralgia and haematuria. He is admitted to the local hospital where investigations reveal deranged renal function and a raised serum IgA.

14. THEME: CRYOGLOBULINAEMIA AND RENAL FAILURE

A   Epstein–Barr virus
B   Hepatitis B virus
C   Infective endocarditis
D   Leptospirosis
E   Lymphoma
F   Malaria
G   Multiple myeloma
H   Rheumatoid arthritis
I   Sjögren's syndrome
J   Waldenström's macroglobulinaemia

The patients below have all presented with renal failure and cryoglobulinaemia. Please choose the most appropriate diagnosis from the above list. Each diagnosis may be used once, more than once or not at all.

1. A 31-year-old woman with a known symmetrical erosive polyarthropathy and anti-Ro and anti-La antibodies presents with a severe vasculitic rash of the hands and feet. Subsequent investigations reveal: Na$^+$ 131 mmol/l, K$^+$ 6.3 mmol/l, urea 19.6 mmol/l, and creatinine 509 μmol/l.

2. A 26-year-old canoeist presents to the Emergency Department 2 weeks after a flu-like illness associated with a headache, myalgia and malaise. On examination, he is jaundiced and has tender hepatosplenomegaly. Investigations reveal: haemoglobin 8.4 g/dl, MCV 101.2 fl, WCC 14.8 × 10^9/l, platelets 400 × 10^9/l; Na$^+$ 134 mmol/l, K$^+$ 5.8 mmol/l, urea 15.6 mmol/l, and creatinine 388 μmol/l. Over the next 24 hours he develops a rash over his lower limbs.

3. A 61-year-old man with a history of childhood rheumatic fever presents to the Emergency Department with a vasculitic rash, increasing peripheral oedema and dyspnoea. On examination, he is anaemic and has a temperature of 38.5 °C. He has a harsh pansystolic murmur at the apex and is in quite marked bilateral ventricular failure. He also has a vasculitic rash affecting his hands and feet.

4. A 16-year-old schoolboy develops a sore throat, associated with lethargy and malaise. He has markedly swollen glands in the neck and under his arms and in the last 24 hours has developed a rash over his feet. Subsequent investigations reveal atypical mononuclear cells in the blood.

5. A 73-year-old man is referred to Medical Out-patients with a 3-month history of increasing lethargy and weight loss. Investigations reveal a normochromic, normocytic anaemia with rouleaux formation. His corrected Ca^{2+} is 2.32 mmol/l; ESR 130 mm/h. Plasma electrophoresis confirms an IgM paraproteinaemia; bone marrow aspirate shows lymphoplasmacytoid cells. There are no lytic lesions seen in any of his radiographs.

15. THEME: NEPHROTOXIC DRUGS

A   Amphotericin B
B   Co-trimoxazole
C   Diclofenac
D   Gentamicin
E   Gold
F   Lithium
G   Penicillamine
H   Penicillin
I   Perindopril
J   Tetracycline

The patients below have all presented with renal failure secondary to their medications. Please choose the most appropriate cause from the above list. Each option may be used once, more than once or not at all.

1. A 29-year-old man is being treated in hospital for acute myeloid leukaemia (AML). He has developed severe oral and oesophageal candidiasis and is started on intravenous therapy. One week later routine blood tests reveal: Na+ 132 mmol/l, K+ 5.9 mmol/l, urea 32 mmol/l and creatinine 550 μmol/l.

2. A 67-year-old woman is being treated for Gram-negative sepsis with intravenous antibiotics. She is clinically a lot better, although in the last few days her renal function has started to deteriorate and she complains of hearing loss.

3. A 22-year-old woman with poorly controlled rheumatoid arthritis is admitted with worsening peripheral oedema and oliguria. She has recently been started on injections of a new therapy. Her U&Es are: Na+ 130 mmol/l, K+ 6.9 mmol/l, urea 52 mmol/l and creatinine 1050 μmol/l.

4. An 85-year-old man with known peripheral vascular disease is admitted with an acute anterior myocardial infarction (MI) and left ventricular failure (LVF). He is started on several 'prognosis-changing' therapies and makes a relatively unremarkable recovery. On review in the Out-patients' Department, however, he complains of a dry, irritating cough and severe malaise. Examination of his cardiovascular and respiratory systems is unremarkable. His U&Es show: Na+ 129 mmol/l, K+ 6.4 mmol/l, urea 23 mmol/l, and creatinine 500 μmol/l.

5. A 23-year-old, HIV-positive man is admitted with a 5-day history of fever and a dry cough. He is started on treatment for an 'atypical' pneumonia. Several days later his renal function has deteriorated dramatically although his chest infection has improved.

16. THEME: RENAL MANIFESTATIONS OF SYSTEMIC DISEASE

A   Crohn's disease
B   Diabetes mellitus
C   Hepatitis B
D   Hepatitis C
E   Mixed connective tissue disease
F   Multiple myeloma
G   Sarcoidosis
H   Sickle-cell disease
I   Systemic lupus erythematosus
J   Systemic sclerosis

The patients below have all presented with renal complications of a systemic disease. Please choose the most appropriate diagnosis from the above list. Each diagnosis may be used once, more than once or not at all.

1. A 25-year-old Afro-Caribbean man presents to the Emergency Department with a 48-hour history of pains in the legs, abdomen and back, associated with frank haematuria. Subsequent investigations reveal: haemoglobin 6.1 g/dl, WCC 14.3×10^9/l, platelets 498×10^9/l; Na^+ 131 mmol/l, K^+ 3.9 mmol/l, urea 14.7 mmol/l and creatinine 110 μmol/l.

2. A 37-year-old woman with known pulmonary infiltrates and bilateral hilar lymphadenopathy on her chest radiograph presents to her GP with malaise and lethargy. Routine investigations reveal: haemoglobin 7.5 g/dl, WCC 4.8×10^9/l, platelets 322×10^9/l; Na^+ 129 mmol/l, K^+ 5.9 mmol/l, urea 32 mmol/l and creatinine 650 μmol/l.

3. An 18-year-old woman with a malar rash and arthritis presents to her GP with increasing malaise, associated with facial and ankle oedema. Of note, her BP is 210/100 mmHg and urinalysis shows proteinuria +++, blood +, nitrites and leucocytes both negative.

4. A 39-year-old man presents to the Emergency Department with severe left-sided abdominal pain associated with fever and haematuria. On examination, he has a temperature of 39.5 °C and is noted to have multiple mouth ulcers. Abdominal examination reveals multiple fistulae and scars, with left loin tenderness. Urinalysis shows: blood ++, protein +, leucocytes +++, nitrites negative. The chest and abdominal radiographs show no signs of obstruction or perforation.

5. A 29-year-old previous intravenous drug user presents to his GP with a 2-week history of swollen ankles, haematuria and poor urine output. After admission to hospital, investigations reveal a nephrotic syndrome secondary to type I mesangiocapillary nephritis. Blood tests reveal an RNA virus-positive hepatitis.

17. THEME: URINARY INCONTINENCE

A   Benign prostatic hypertrophy
B   Cystocoele
C   Detrusor instability
D   Diuretic therapy
E   Immobility
F   Multiple sclerosis
G   Normal-pressure hydrocephalus
H   Radiation cystitis
I   Spinal cord compression
J   Urinary tract infection

The patients below have all presented with urinary incontinence. Please choose the most likely diagnosis from the above list. Each diagnosis may be used once, more than once or not at all.

1. A 57-year-old woman with metastatic carcinoma of the breast presents to the Emergency Department with urinary incontinence, constipation and weakness in her lower limbs. On examination, she has a palpable bladder and a sensory level defined at T10.

2. An 87-year-old man presents to the Medicine for the Elderly Out-patients' Clinic with increasing confusion, falls and incontinence. On examination he has an AMTS of 5/10 and gait dyspraxia. Urinalysis is unremarkable.

3. A 79-year-old man with a previous history of a transurethral resection of prostate (TURP) presents to his GP with increasing urinary incontinence associated with urgency and frequency. Routine bloods, including U&Es and PSA, are normal and urinalysis is unremarkable. His symptoms improve dramatically with oxybutynin.

4. A 66-year-old man presents to his GP with increasing urinary incontinence associated with frequency, poor stream and terminal dribbling. His PSA is 2.1 nmol/l. His symptoms improve with terazosin.

5. A 91-year-old woman who is normally fit and well presents to the Emergency Department with increasing confusion and falls. Urinalysis shows: blood ++, protein ++, nitrites +.

18. THEME: URINARY TRACT OBSTRUCTION I

A   Benign prostatic hypertrophy
B   Myelomatous light chains
C   Neurogenic bladder
D   Prostatic carcinoma
E   Renal stones
F   Retroperitoneal fibrosis
G   Sickle-cell disease
H   Squamous-cell carcinoma of the bladder
I   Transitional-cell carcinoma of the bladder
J   Ureteric stricture

The patients below have all presented with urinary tract obstruction. Please choose the most appropriate diagnosis from the above list. Each diagnosis may be used once, more than once or not at all.

1. A 39-year-old woman with recurrent *Proteus* urinary tract infections and loin pain presents with dysuria, haematuria and oliguria for the past 4 days. Investigations show: Na^+ 131 mmol/l, K^+ 5.3 mmol/l, urea 25.6 mmol/l and creatinine 213 μmol/l. Her abdominal radiograph reveals a large calcified mass in the left side of the abdomen and an ultrasound scan shows a hydronephrotic left kidney.

2. A 69-year-old man presents to the Emergency Department with pain in his thoracolumbar spine and left-sided ribs. He has had increasing urinary frequency, poor stream and terminal dribbling for several months. On examination, he is tender over his lower thoracic spine and the anterior aspects of his fifth to seventh ribs. He has a palpable bladder. Neurological examination of the lower limbs is normal.

3. A 71-year-old woman presents in the Emergency Department with jaundice and oliguria for 10 days, associated with a 3-month history of vague abdominal pain. An ultrasound scan confirms a large mass in the head of the pancreas, and bilateral hydroureters and hydronephrosis.

4. A 79-year-old man presents to the Emergency Department with a 3-month history of back pain, now associated with confusion and constipation. Investigations reveal: ESR 132 mm/h and corrected Ca^{2+} 3.23 mmol/l. Lytic lesions are seen in his ribs and proximal left femur on radiography.

5. A 45-year-old woman presents to her GP with progressive blurring of her vision, falls and difficulty in passing urine. On examination, she has weakness in both lower limbs with a sensory level at T10 and a palpable bladder. The GP also notices a large mass in her left breast.

19. THEME: URINARY TRACT OBSTRUCTION II

A   Automatic bladder
B   Benign prostatic hypertrophy
C   Bladder carcinoma
D   Clot retention
E   Constipation
F   Neurogenic bladder
G   Prostatic carcinoma
H   Prostatic oedema
I   Urethral stricture
J   External sphincter dyssynergia

The patients below have all presented with retention of urine. Please select the most appropriate diagnosis from the above list. Each diagnosis may be used once, more than once or not at all.

1. A 75-year-old man presents to his GP with a 2-year history of increasing hesitancy in starting to void, lessened force and terminal dribbling. Abdominal examination is unremarkable. Rectal examination reveals a smoothly enlarged prostate. His U&Es include: urea 7.2 mmol/l, creatinine 99 μmol/l; his PSA is 8 nmol/l.

2. A 60-year-old man with a long history of type 2 diabetes presents complaining of incontinence of urine and faeces. He has no abdominal pain or other symptoms other than those associated with diabetes (peripheral neuropathy, retinopathy). On examination, a non-tender mass is felt in the lower abdomen, which is dull to percussion, arises from the pelvis and extends almost to the umbilicus. Rectal examination reveals a normal-sized prostate. Urethral catheterisation drains 1500 ml of urine. His U&Es include: urea 15.2 mmol/l, creatinine 190 μmol/l; and his PSA is less than 4 nmol/l.

3. A 60 year old man who is known to have inoperable bladder cancer is admitted with acute urinary retention. On direct questioning, he admits to noticing several previous episodes of frank blood in his urine over the past few months. Today he again describes frank haematuria. On rectal examination, the prostate gland feels normal in size. A urinary catheter drains approximately 400 ml of deeply bloodstained urine, then stops working. His U&Es include: urea 9.1 mmol/l, creatinine 127 μmol/l; his PSA is less than 4 nmol/l.

4. A 42-year-old man undergoes a difficult recurrent left inguino-scrotal hernia repair. Post-operatively, the FY1 doctor is asked to review the patient, who is complaining of increasingly severe lower abdominal pain. On examination, a tender mass is felt in the lower abdomen which is dull to percussion, arises from the pelvis and extends almost to the umbilicus. Rectal examination reveals a normal-sized prostate. His U&Es include: urea 9.2 mmol/l, creatinine 104 μmol/l; his PSA is less than 4 nmol/l.

5. You are asked to review a 26-year-old man with spina bifida who has had a long-term indwelling urethral catheter. He has presented to the Emergency Department with a blocked catheter that has been removed. You are called because the charge nurse is unable to replace the catheter. On attempted insertion, you are unable to pass the catheter more than 1 cm into the urethra. Further attempts cause bleeding from the urethral meatus.

20. THEME: SCROTAL SWELLINGS

A   Acute haematocele
B   Acute epididymo-orchitis
C   Epididymal cyst
D   Idiopathic (primary) hydrocele
E   Inguinal hernia
F   Testicular seminoma
G   Testicular teratoma
H   Testicular torsion
I   Tuberculous orchitis
J   Varicocele

The patients below have all presented with hemiscrotal swellings. Please select the most appropriate diagnosis from the above list. Each diagnosis may be used once, more than once or not at all.

1. A 49-year-old man presented to his GP complaining of a gradually enlarging painless swelling of his left scrotum, big enough to cause him social embarrassment. On examination, the left scrotum was swollen, non-tender, fluctuant and transilluminable. The testis was impalpable and the scrotal neck normal.

2. A 12-year-old boy presented to the Emergency Department with a sudden onset of severe right scrotal pain and vomiting. On examination the right testis was swollen and hanging higher than the left. Skin colour was normal. The testis on the right was so tender to palpation that the child refused careful examination of the hemiscrotal contents.

3. A 22-year-old man presented to his GP with swelling of his left hemiscrotum. He had experienced some dull aching in the scrotum and had been feeling generally unwell for several weeks. The left testis was slightly enlarged and felt hard and irregular in shape. Blood tests showed raised α-fetoprotein (α-FP) and β-human chorionic gonadotrophin (β-hCG).

4. A 30-year-old man was seen in the Emergency Department complaining of 2 days of increasingly severe right scrotal pain and swelling. Direct questioning revealed some frequency of micturition and dysuria for several days. On examination, he was febrile (39 °C) and the right hemiscrotum was swollen and tender. The overlying skin was red and hot. Urine dipstix testing showed: leucocytes +++, nitrite +; the WCC was 16.8 × 10⁹/l.

5. A 25-year-old man presented via the Emergency Department complaining of a tender right scrotal swelling. He gave a history of a football injury 2 days ago, which had caused him some discomfort, followed by rapid onset of swelling and pain yesterday. On examination, the right hemiscrotum was tense, tender and fluctuant and did not transilluminate. The testis could not be palpated.

21. THEME: MENORRHAGIA

A   Adenomyosis
B   Endometrial polyp
C   Fibroids
D   Hypothyroidism
E   Intrauterine contraceptive device
F   Pelvic inflammatory disease
G   Physiological
H   Salpingitis
I   Thrombocytopenia
J   von Willebrand's disease

The patients below have all presented with menorrhagia. Please choose the most appropriate diagnosis from the above list. Each diagnosis may be used once, more than once or not at all.

1. A 29-year-old woman presents to her GP with an 18-month history of worsening, painless menorrhagia. She is being forced to take 2-3 days off work per month, because the bleeding is so heavy. On examination, she is clinically anaemic and has a slightly enlarged, bulky uterus.

2. A 34-year-old woman presents to her GP with an 8-month history of severe menorrhagia and lower abdominal pain. On examination, she has a tender, enlarged uterus, equivalent to a 16-week pregnancy. She has a total abdominal hysterectomy and the subsequent pathology report confirms 'a fibromyomatous reaction with endometrial tissue within the myometrium continuous with the normal endometrium'.

3. A 25-year-old woman presents to her GP 3 months after stopping the oral contraceptive pill. Over the last 2 months her periods have become 'extremely heavy and prolonged'. On further questioning, she has vaginal bleeding for 4-5 days and does not appear to use excessive numbers of tampons or pads. Examination, including speculum and bimanual examinations, are unremarkable. The FBC results are: haemoglobin 12.3 g/dl, MCV 89 fl, WCC 4.9 × 10^9/l, and platelets 316 × 10^9/l. The clotting screen shows a normal bleeding time and an activated partial thromboplastin time (APTT) of 35 seconds.

4. A 21-year-old woman, previously treated for a chlamydial urethritis, presents to her GP with pelvic pain and menorrhagia. The results from an endocervical smear confirm the presence of *Chlamydia trachomatis*.

5. A 16-year-old student presents to her GP with increasingly heavy periods and fatigue. Subsequent investigations reveal: haemoglobin 8.9 g/dl, MCV 69 fl, WCC 6.5 × 10^9/l, platelets 277 × 10^9/l; bleeding time prolonged, APTT 54 seconds.

22. THEME: INTERMENSTRUAL BLEEDING

A Cervical carcinoma
B Cervical ectropion
C Cervical polyp
D Dysfunctional uterine bleeding
E Ectopic pregnancy
F Endometrial carcinoma
G Endometriosis
H Intrauterine contraceptive device
I Threatened abortion
J Vaginitis

The patients below have all presented with intermenstrual bleeding. Please choose the most appropriate diagnosis from the above list. Each diagnosis may be used once, more than once or not at all.

1. A 37-year-old woman presents to her GP with a 2-month history of post-coital bleeding. On speculum examination there is an ulcerated, friable lesion of the cervix. An endocervical smear confirms the presence of 'abnormal cells with dyskaryotic nuclei'.

2. A 31-year-old woman presents to her GP with irregular periods, deep dyspareunia, dysmenorrhoea and intermenstrual bleeding. The diagnosis is confirmed on laparoscopy and improves after diathermy and subsequent danazol.

3. A 46-year-old nulliparous woman presents to her GP with irregular periods and intermenstrual bleeding. Subsequent hysteroscopy and biopsy confirms the presence of a poorly differentiated adenocarcinoma.

4. A 26-year-old woman presents to her GP with a 4-month history of post-coital and intermenstrual bleeding. On speculum examination the cervix is noted to be everted and 'ulcerated'. Her smear is subsequently reported as normal.

5. A 32-year-old woman with no previous menstrual problems presents in the Emergency Department with severe right-sided lower abdominal pain and vaginal bleeding, 7 weeks after her last normal period. Her β-human chorionic gonadotrophin (β-hCG) test is positive and emergency ultrasound scan confirms 'no gestational sac seen within the uterus'.

23. THEME: SECONDARY AMENORRHOEA

A   Adrenal carcinoma
B   Anorexia nervosa
C   Congenital adrenal hyperplasia
D   Cushing's syndrome
E   Hypothalamic infarction
F   Hypothyroidism
G   Panhypopituitarism
H   Polycystic ovary syndrome
I   Pregnancy
J   Prolactinoma

The patients below have all presented with secondary amenorrhoea. Please choose the most appropriate diagnosis from the above list. Each diagnosis may be used once, more than once or not at all.

1. A previously fit and well 23-year-old woman presents to her GP with a 9-month history of amenorrhoea and galactorrhoea. Examination is remarkable only for expressible galactorrhoea. Her β-hCG is negative. Subsequent CT head scan shows a 0.6-cm mass in the left side of the pituitary gland. Her 9-am cortisol is 550 nmol/l, prolactin 2824 mU/l.   J

2. A 26-year-old woman presents to her GP with obesity, hirsutism and secondary amenorrhoea. Investigations reveal a raised serum luteinising hormone (LH) and testosterone, and low sex hormone-binding globulin (SHBG). Her serum prolactin is 645 mU/l.   H

3. A previously fit and well, 24-year-old woman presents to her GP with gross weight loss and amenorrhoea for 4 months. Examination is unremarkable other than her obvious weight loss. Her BMI is 15 kg/m². Investigations reveal: haemoglobin 10.5 g/dl, MCV 103 fl, WCC 4.1×10^9/l, platelets 198×10^9/l; Na⁺ 134 mmol/l, K⁺ 3.9 mmol/l, urea 2.7 mmol/l, creatinine 72 μmol/l; total bilirubin 12 μmol/l, AST 23 IU/l, ALT 24 IU/l, albumin 31 g/l; red cell folate low.   B

4. A 16-year-old schoolgirl presents to her GP with oligomenorrhoea for 4 months, and amenorrhoea for the past 2 months. On examination, she has a short stature and hirsutism but otherwise examination is unremarkable. Subsequent investigations confirm high serum and urinary 17α-hydroxyprogesterone.   C

5. A 36-year-old woman presents to her GP 4 months after the complicated delivery of her last baby. She suffered a large post-partum haemorrhage, requiring operative intervention and a 7-unit blood transfusion. She had been unable to breastfeed and has subsequently not had a period. She feels extremely weak, lethargic and generally 'washed out'.   G   E

24. THEME: PRURITUS VULVAE

A Atopic eczema
B Candidiasis
C Diabetes mellitus
D Gonorrhoea
E Pubic lice
F Trichomoniasis
G Urinary incontinence
H Vaginal warts
I Vulval carcinoma
J Vulval dystrophy

The patients below have all presented with pruritus vulvae. Please choose the most appropriate diagnosis from the above list. Each scenario may have more than one correct answer.

1. A 32-year-old woman presents to her GP, 6 weeks after a 'one night stand' with a work colleague. She has developed intense itching around the vagina and has developed several small lesions on her labia. A speculum examination and subsequent smear result are both normal. ☐

2. A 23-year-old woman presents to her GP with pruritus around the vulva and a vaginal discharge. Examination, including vaginal speculum examination, is remarkable only for the pruritus marks around the vulva and an offensive vaginal discharge. Subsequent microbiology results confirm the presence of Gram-negative diplococcus. ☐

3. A 51-year-old woman presents to her GP with intense pruritus around the vulva. On examination, she is well and her capillary blood glucose is 4.9 mmol/l. The vulva is seen to be atrophic, flat and shiny but speculum examination is unremarkable. A small biopsy confirms 'hypoplastic areas with no evidence of atypia'. The condition improves with oestrogen cream. ☐

4. A 19-year-old woman presents to her GP with an offensive vaginal discharge and pruritus vulvae. On examination, she is seen to have a frothy, green discharge, erythema of the vulva and punctate haemorrhages of the cervix. Subsequent microbiology results confirm the presence of 'pear-shaped flagellate protozoans'. ☐

5. A 49-year-old obese woman presents to her GP with pruritus vulvae and a creamy vaginal discharge. On examination, she is obese and her capillary blood glucose is 11.8 mmol/l. Gynaecological examination is remarkable only for white membranous patches over the vulva and the vaginal discharge. Subsequent investigations confirm an Hb A_{1c} of 10.9% and 'Gram-positive yeast cells with pseudohyphae' in the discharge. ☐

25. THEME: NEOPLASMS OF THE FEMALE GENITAL TRACT

A Adenocarcinoma
B Brenner tumour
C Dysgerminoma
D Hydatidiform mole
E Leiomyoma
F Mature cystic teratoma
G Mucinous cystadenoma
H Papillary serous cystadenocarcinoma
I Squamous-cell carcinoma
J Thecoma

For each of the women below, select the most likely neoplasm from the above list. Each tumour may be used once, more than once or not at all.

1. A 26-year-old woman presents with a long history of abdominal and pelvic pain. Investigations show a left-sided cystic ovarian mass measuring 10 cm in diameter. The excised mass has a smooth external surface. Slicing reveals a unilocular cyst filled with sebaceous material and matted hair. Areas of bone and a tooth are also visible.

2. A 65-year-old woman presents with post-menopausal bleeding. She is nulliparous, overweight and hypertensive. Histological examination of an endometrial aspirate shows a malignant tumour composed of closely packed glands with a small amount of mucin formation.

3. A 72-year-old woman presents with vulval itching and soreness. On examination, she has a 3-cm ulcer with raised, rolled, everted edges on the right labium majus. She also has enlarged lymph nodes in the right groin. Biopsy of the ulcer edge shows a malignant tumour composed of eosinophilic cells, with keratin pearl formation.

4. A 42-year-old woman presents with abdominal pain and distension. On examination, an abdominal mass is palpable below the umbilicus. Ultrasound shows multiple masses in the body of the uterus suggestive of 'fibroids'. Naked eye examination of the hysterectomy specimen shows several well-circumscribed intramyometrial masses with a white, whorled cut surface. Histology of the masses shows benign mesenchymal neoplasms.

5. A 23-year-old woman presents with a large, right-sided, solid ovarian mass. The excised mass has a smooth external surface. Histological examination shows a germ-cell tumour composed of large polygonal cells with prominent nucleoli. Numerous lymphocytes are also present.

CHAPTER 3

Musculoskeletal

1. THEME: CUTANEOUS INNERVATION OF THE UPPER LIMB

A   Anterior interosseus nerve
B   Axillary nerve
C   Medial cutaneous nerve of the forearm
D   Median nerve
E   Musculocutaneous nerve
F   Posterior cutaneous nerve of the arm
G   Posterior cutaneous nerve of the forearm
H   Posterior interosseus nerve
I   Radial nerve
J   Ulnar nerve

For each of the options below, identify the innervation of the skin from the above list. Each nerve may be used once, more than once or not at all.

1. Distal attachment of the deltoid muscle.   B

2. Medial epicondyle of the humerus.   J

3. Scaphoid fossa.   I

4. Thenar eminence.   D

5. Nail bed of the little finger.   G

2. THEME: NERVE SUPPLY OF THE MUSCLES OF THE UPPER LIMB

A   Anterior interosseus nerve
B   Axillary nerve
C   Long thoracic nerve
D   Lower subscapular nerve
E   Medial cutaneous nerve of the forearm
F   Median nerve
G   Musculocutaneous nerve
H   Posterior interosseus nerve
I   Radial nerve
J   Ulnar nerve

For each of the muscles below, identify its nerve supply from the above list. Each nerve may be used once, more than once or not at all.

1. Teres major.

2. Brachioradialis.

3. Supinator.

4. Flexor carpi ulnaris.

5. Flexor carpi radialis.

3. THEME: MUSCLE ATTACHMENTS OF THE FOREARM

A   Biceps
B   Brachialis
C   Brachioradialis
D   Deltoid
E   Extensor carpi radialis brevis
F   Flexor carpi ulnaris
G   Flexor digitorum profundus
H   Flexor pollicis longus
I   Pronator teres
J   Supinator
K   Triceps

For each of the bony attachments below, choose the most appropriate muscle from the above list. Each muscle may be used once, more than once or not at all.

1. Lateral supracondylar ridge of the humerus. ☐

2. Olecranon process of the ulna. ☐

3. Anterior aspect of the lateral epicondyle of the humerus. ☐

4. Coronoid process of the ulna. ☐

5. Proximal anterior surface of the radius. ☐

4. THEME: RELATIONSHIPS OF THE UPPER LIMB

A   Anterior interosseus nerve
B   Biceps tendon
C   Brachial artery
D   Common interosseus artery
E   Median nerve
F   Posterior interosseus nerve
G   Radial artery
H   Radial nerve
I   Ulnar artery
J   Ulnar nerve

For each of the anatomical descriptions below, choose the most appropriate structure from the above list. Each structure may be used once, more than once or not at all.

1. Lies in contact with the posterior shaft of the humerus. G ☐

2. Lies in contact with the posterior surface of the medial epicondyle of the humerus.   ☐

3. Passes between the two heads of pronator teres.   ☐

4. Divides at the level of the neck of the radius.   ☐

5. Passes between the heads of the first palmar interosseus muscles.   ☐

5. THEME: CUTANEOUS INNERVATION OF THE LOWER LIMB

A   Deep peroneal (anterior tibial) nerve
B   Genitofemoral nerve
C   Intermediate cutaneous nerve of the thigh
D   Lateral cutaneous nerve of the thigh
E   Medial cutaneous nerve of the thigh
F   Posterior cutaneous nerve of the thigh
G   Posterior tibial nerve
H   Saphenous nerve
I   Superficial peroneal (musculocutaneous) nerve
J   Sural nerve

For each of the options below, identify the innervation of the skin from the above list. Each nerve may be used once, more than once or not at all.

1. Saphenous opening.

2. Greater trochanter.

3. Lower shin.

4. Lateral side of the foot.

5. Dorsal aspect of the first interdigital web.

6. THEME: NERVE SUPPLY OF THE MUSCLES OF THE LOWER LIMB

A   Deep peroneal (anterior tibial) nerve
B   Common peroneal (lateral popliteal) nerve
C   Femoral nerve
D   Inferior gluteal nerve
E   Medial plantar nerve
F   Obturator nerve
G   Sciatic nerve
H   Superficial peroneal (musculocutaneous) nerve
I   Sural nerve
J   Tibial (posterior tibial) nerve

For each of the muscles below, identify its nerve supply from the above list. Each nerve may be used once, more than once or not at all.

1. Adductor longus.

2. Biceps.

3. Extensor digitorum longus.

4. Peroneus brevis.

5. Tibialis posterior.

7. THEME: RELATIONSHIPS OF THE LOWER LIMB

A   Anterior tibial artery
B   Common peroneal nerve
C   Femoral artery
D   Femoral nerve
E   Great saphenous vein
F   Peroneal artery
G   Posterior tibial artery
H   Sciatic nerve
I   Small saphenous vein
J   Tibial nerve

For each of the anatomical descriptions below, choose the most appropriate structure from the above list. Each structure may be used once, more than once or not at all.

1. Passes through the saphenous opening in the fascia lata. ☐

2. Passes through the opening in the adductor magnus tendon. ☐

3. Is closely related to the lateral aspect of the neck of the fibula. ☐

4. Lies medial to the talus. ☐

5. Lies anterior to the lateral malleolus. ☐

8. THEME: MUSCLE ATTACHMENTS OF THE LOWER LIMB

A   Adductor longus
B   Adductor magnus
C   Biceps femoris
D   Peroneus brevis
E   Peroneus longus
F   Rectus femoris
G   Semimembranosus
H   Soleus
I   Tibialis anterior
J   Tibialis posterior

For each of the bony attachments below, choose the most appropriate muscle from the above list. Each muscle may be used once, more than once or not at all.

1. The anterior inferior iliac spine.

2. The body of the pubis.

3. The head of the fibula.

4. The medial cuneiform bone.

5. The styloid process of the fifth metatarsal.

9. THEME: COMPLICATIONS OF FRACTURES

A Algodystrophy (Sudeck's atrophy)
B Avascular necrosis
C Compartment syndrome
D Delayed union
E Malunion
F Nerve injury
G Non-union
H Myositis ossificans
I Osteoarthritis
J Vascular injury

The patients below have all sustained injuries resulting in fractures. Please select the most likely fracture complication from the above list. Each complication may be used once, more than once or not at all.

1. A 10-year-old child fell onto her outstretched hand 6 hours ago. The child is complaining of severe pain that was initially in the elbow but is now more severe in the forearm. Both areas are swollen and tender. Examination reveals a palpable rapid pulse, but decreased sensation in the hand with reduced capillary return.

2. A 36-year-old computer programmer fell onto his outstretched hand and subsequently developed a painful wrist. An initial visit to the Emergency Department resulted in a normal radiograph and his discharge. He was still complaining of pain 10 months later, however, and again attended the Emergency Department. A further radiograph was performed and the attending Emergency Department officer informed him that he had an 'abnormal extra bone in the wrist'.

3. A 27-year-old footballer had a marked deformity of the knee after a hard tackle. He subsequently attended the Emergency Department, where the deformity was immediately reduced by the orthopaedic team. He still has marked swelling and pain of the knee, but also now has reduced sensation on the dorsum of the foot, with an associated foot drop. The foot pulses are present.

4. A 60-year-old woman falls on her outstretched hand. There is tenderness and a deformity at the wrist, in which the hand is displaced backwards and over to the radial side. Three months later she complains of continuous burning pain and swelling in the hand.

5. A 56-year-old violinist tripped and suffered an injury to his right wrist. He subsequently underwent operative treatment for a comminuted fracture of the distal radius and ulna. The outcome of surgery was said to be satisfactory and he returned to concert performance 6 months later. Four years later he complains of increasing pain and swelling in the wrist and becomes unable to continue in his career.

10. THEME: UPPER LIMB INJURIES

A   Acromioclavicular joint dislocation
B   Colles' fracture
C   Dislocated shoulder
D   Fracture of the clavicle
E   Fracture of the proximal humerus
F   Fracture of the radial head
G   Fracture of the shaft of the humerus
H   Scaphoid fracture
I   Smith's fracture
J   Supracondylar fracture of the humerus

The patients below have all fallen, injuring their upper limb. Please select the most appropriate fracture or dislocation from the above list. Each injury may be used once, more than once or not at all.

1. A 20-year-old man falls on his backward-stretching hand. He is supporting his arm with his opposite hand. The lateral outline of the shoulder is flattened and a small bulge is seen and felt just below the clavicle. There is a small area of anaesthesia over the distal attachment of the deltoid muscle.

2. A 70-year-old woman falls on her elbow. She has marked bruising and tenderness of the upper arm. Neurovascular examination reveals a wrist drop.

3. A 24-year-old man presents 3 months after spraining his wrist, when he fell on his outstretched hand. He complains of persistent pain and weakness in the wrist.

4. A 10-year-old child fell onto his outstretched hand 30 minutes ago. The child is complaining of severe pain in the elbow, which is very swollen and tender. Examination reveals an absent radial pulse.

5. A 31-year-old merchant banker fell from his horse onto his outstretched hand while hunting in Kent. He attends the Emergency Department the following day complaining of pain and decreased movement of the elbow. A radiograph of the elbow was reported as showing an effusion of the elbow joint with a 'fat pad sign' but no obvious fracture. Several weeks later the patient continues to complain of loss of extension at the elbow.

11. THEME: MONOARTHRITIS

A   Candidiasis
B   Charcot's joint
C   Gonococcal arthritis
D   Gout
E   Haemarthrosis
F   Osteoarthritis
G   Pyrophosphate arthritis
H   Reiter's syndrome
I   Staphylococcal arthritis
J   Tuberculous arthritis

The following patients have all presented with a monoarthritis. Please choose the most appropriate diagnosis from the above list. Each diagnosis may be used once, more than once or not at all.

1. A 43-year-old publican presents to his GP with a 24-hour history of an 'exquisitely tender' right big toe. On examination, he is in obvious distress but is otherwise well. The interphalangeal joint of his right big toe is hot, red and very tender. Joint aspiration reveals no organisms but negatively birefringent crystals under polarised light.

2. An 84-year-old man presents to his GP with an acutely swollen left knee. Subsequent investigations reveal intra-articular calcification on the radiographs and joint aspiration reveals positively birefringent crystals under polarised light.

3. A 27-year-old man presents to the Emergency Department with an acutely swollen and painful right knee associated with 'red, gritty eyes' and dysuria. He has recently returned from South-East Asia, where he had diarrhoea and vomiting for several days.

4. A 61-year-old man with long-standing diabetes mellitus presents to the Emergency Department acutely unwell. A diagnosis of lobar pneumonia is made and he is admitted. The man incidentally is found to have a swollen, grossly deformed left ankle, associated with signs of a peripheral sensory neuropathy.

5. A 71-year-old woman with a chronic arthritis presents to the Emergency Department with an acutely painful, hot and swollen left shoulder 3 days after her GP had given her an intra-articular steroid injection.

12. THEME: POLYARTHRITIS

A   Behçet's syndrome
B   Inflammatory bowel disease
C   Osteoarthritis
D   Psoriasis
E   Rheumatic fever
F   Rheumatoid arthritis
G   Rubella
H   Sjögren's syndrome
I   Still's disease
J   Systemic lupus erythematosus

The following patients have all presented with a polyarthritis. Please choose the most appropriate diagnosis from the above list. Each diagnosis may be used once, more than once or not at all.

1. A 36-year-old man presents to his GP with increasing swelling and pain in the proximal interphalangeal joints of both hands. Several of the joints are deformed and the fingers show ulnar deviation. He is noted to have a scaly plaque on his left elbow and in his hairline.

2. A 65-year-old woman presents to her GP with increasing pain and swelling of her left knee, associated with decreasing mobility. Examination reveals a swollen, painful left knee, associated with an asymmetrical arthropathy of the distal interphalangeal joints of her hands.

3. A 21-year-old man, originally from a Mediterranean coastal town, presents to his GP with ulceration affecting his mouth and scrotum. He also complains of painful, swollen ankles, knees and right elbow. He has had several similar attacks in the past, some associated with diarrhoea and vomiting.

4. A 17-year-old student presents to her GP with a rash over her cheeks and pain and swelling in her hands and feet. Routine investigations reveal anti-double-stranded DNA (anti-dsDNA) antibodies.

5. A 43-year-old woman with a long-standing arthritis presents to her GP with itchy eyes and a dry mouth. Investigations reveal a positive Schirmer's test and anti-Ro and anti-La antibodies.

13. THEME: COMPLICATIONS OF RHEUMATOID ARTHRITIS

A   Episcleritis
B   Felty's syndrome
C   Mononeuritis multiplex
D   Pericardial effusion
E   Pericarditis
F   Peripheral sensory neuropathy
G   Pleural effusion
H   Pulmonary fibrosis
I   Scleromalacia
J   Sjögren's syndrome

The following patients have all presented with complications of their rheumatoid disease. Please choose the most appropriate diagnosis from the above list. Each diagnosis may be used once, more than once or not at all.

1. A 42-year-old woman with known rheumatoid arthritis presents to her GP with episodes of tripping over her right foot and numbness in her left hand. On examination, she has an obvious right foot drop and wasting of the thenar eminence associated with sensory loss over the radial two and a half fingers of the hand.

2. A 37-year-old man with long-standing rheumatoid arthritis presents to the Emergency Department with left-sided chest pain. On examination, he has a temperature of 37.8 °C and a 'squeaky' murmur over the apex beat. The electrocardiograpm (ECG) reveals saddle-shaped ST elevation in leads V_1, V_4 and V_5, I and aVF.

3. A 41-year-old man with long-standing rheumatoid arthritis presents to his GP with a 5-month history of worsening pins and needles in his hands and feet.

4. A 47-year-old woman with rheumatoid arthritis presents with a 2-day history of painful, red eyes. On examination, her visual acuity is normal but she is obviously distressed and there is marked dilatation of the deep and superficial scleral vessels.

5. A 36-year-old man with long-standing rheumatoid arthritis presents to the Emergency Department with symptoms of an upper respiratory tract infection and lethargy. Examination reveals a mass in the left upper quadrant of the abdomen and a purpuric rash. The U&Es and LFTs are normal but his FBC shows: haemoglobin 8.7 g/dl, MCV 87 fl, WCC 2.8×10^9/l, platelets 34×10^9/l.

14. THEME: DRUGS USED IN RHEUMATOID ARTHRITIS

A   Anti-tumour necrosis factor (TNFα) therapy
B   Azathioprine
C   Celecoxib
D   Diclofenac
E   D-Penicillamine
F   Gold
G   Hydroxychloroquine
H   Methotrexate
I   Prednisolone
J   Sulfasalazine

The following patients have all presented with side-effects of their rheumatoid medications. Please choose the most appropriate cause from the above list. Each option may be used once, more than once or not at all.

1. A 42-year-old woman with long-standing rheumatoid arthritis presents to her GP with severe bruising of the upper and lower limbs. She is noted to have a 'moon face' and centripetal obesity. Her platelet count and clotting screen are both within normal limits.

2. A 25-year-old woman with early rheumatoid arthritis presents to her GP with worsening dyspepsia and a single episode of black, tarry stools 2 weeks previously. She is known to be on a NSAID with a COX index < 0.1.

3. A 36-year-old man with severe rheumatoid arthritis is started on a new agent by the local rheumatologist. He returns to his GP several weeks later complaining that 'his hair is losing its colour and is falling out'. He has also noticed blurred vision. On further questioning, it emerges that the patient has been taking twice the recommended dose.

4. A 29-year-old woman who has recently started on a new agent for her rheumatoid disease presents to her GP with a rash over her cheeks and nose and worsening arthralgia. Routine blood tests reveal: Na$^+$ 131 mmol/l, K$^+$ 5.9 mmol/l, urea 17.9 mmol/l, creatinine 398 μmol/l.

5. A 41-year-old man who is receiving weekly injections for his rheumatoid arthritis presents to his GP with a sore throat associated with a purpuric rash over his torso and upper limbs. He has no signs of meningism or photophobia. An urgent FBC reveals: haemoglobin 6.4 g/dl, MCV 88 fl, WCC 1.0×10^9/l, and platelets 16×10^9/l.

15. THEME: PREDISPOSING FACTORS TO OSTEOARTHROPATHIES

A   Acromegaly
B   Avascular necrosis
C   Congenital dislocation of the hip
D   Ehlers–Danlos syndrome
E   Haemochromatosis
F   Obesity
G   Ochronosis
H   Paget's bone disease
I   Perthes' disease
J   Rheumatoid arthritis

The following patients have all presented with osteoarthritis. Please choose the most appropriate predisposing factor from the above list. Each option may be used once, more than once or not at all.

1. A 49-year-old woman presents to her GP with a 4-month history of pain and swelling of her right knee. She is otherwise systemically well but is noted to be 1.54 m tall and 85 kg in weight.

2. A 79-year old man with a previous left total hip replacement presents to his GP with right hip and knee pain. Routine investigations reveal a normal FBC, U&Es and glucose. The corrected Ca^{2+} is 2.32 mmol/l, PO_4^{3-} 1.05 mmol/l, alkaline phosphatase 432 IU/l. Pelvic radiographs are reported as showing 'increased trabecular pattern and cortical thickening of the right hemipelvis with loss of joint space and osteophyte formation of the right hip'.

3. A 21-year-old Afro-Caribbean man with known sickle-cell disease presents in the Haematology Clinic with left hip pain. Radiographs reveal loss of the right femoral head and periarticular sclerosis.

4. A 23-year old man who works as a contortionist in a travelling circus presents in the Emergency Department with a 6-month history of pain in his left hip. Of note, he has had recurrent dislocations of his shoulders. On examination, he has pain with all movements of the hip and radiographs confirm early osteoarthritic changes.

16. THEME: SERONEGATIVE SPONDYLOARTHROPATHIES

A   Adult Still's disease
B   Ankylosing spondylitis
C   Behçet's syndrome
D   Enteropathic synovitis
E   Psoriasis
F   Reactive arthritis
G   Reiter's syndrome
H   Whipple's disease

The following patients have all presented with a seronegative spondyloarthropathy. Please choose the most appropriate diagnosis from the above list. Each diagnosis may be used once, more than once or not at all.

1. A 59-year-old woman with plaques on the extensor surfaces of her upper limbs presents to her GP with pain in her hands. She has a long-standing deforming arthropathy of her fingers, associated with a telescoping deformity of the right index finger and left little finger.

2. A 42-year-old man presents to his GP with increasing exertional dyspnoea. On examination, he has a characteristic 'question mark' stature with a marked thoracic kyphosis. Respiratory examination reveals some fine inspiratory crepitations at the apices.

3. A 24-year-old man who is being treated for a chlamydial urethritis develops an acutely swollen right knee, associated with painful heels and 'gritty, red eyes'.

4. A 29-year-old man presents to the Emergency Department with severe bloody diarrhoea associated with a painful, swollen left knee and swollen, painful toes. He has been admitted on several occasions over the past few years with similar presentations.

5. A 43-year-old man presents to his GP with a 4-month history of diarrhoea associated with weight loss and pains in the lower back, right hip and some of the small joints of the hand and feet. Gastroenterological investigations reveal periodic acid–Schiff (PAS-)positive macrophages within intestinal biopsies.

17. THEME: REITER'S SYNDROME

A   Achilles' tendonitis
B   Anterior uveitis
C   Arthritis
D   Circinate balanitis
E   Conjunctivitis
F   Keratoderma blennorrhagicum
G   Nail dystrophy
H   Oral ulceration
I   Plantar fasciitis
J   Urethritis

The following patients have all presented with a specific feature(s) of Reiter's syndrome. Please choose the most appropriate feature(s) from the above list. There may be more than one correct answer for each scenario and options may be used more than once

1. A 26-year-old man presents to the Emergency Department with an acute arthritis of his left knee associated with red, 'gritty' eyes and a fever. He is also noted to have ulceration over the glans of his penis.

2. A 14-year-old schoolgirl with a 6-day history of a diarrhoeal illness associated initially with vomiting presents to her GP with the classical triad of Reiter's syndrome and a pigmented rash over her soles and right palm.

3. A 32-year-old man with a 4-day history of a swollen right knee and urethral discharge presents to his GP with blurring of his vision and mild photophobia. The eyes have not been 'sticky' and he has no fever or associated meningism.

4. A 27-year-old woman with recurrent Reiter's syndrome presents to her GP with another acute episode associated with extremely painful ankles, heels and soles.

18. THEME: VASCULITIDES

A   Churg–Strauss syndrome
B   Giant-cell arteritis
C   Henoch–Schönlein purpura
D   Kawasaki's disease
E   Microscopic polyangiitis
F   Polyarteritis nodosa
G   Takayasu's disease
H   Wegener's granulomatosis

The following patients have all presented with a vasculitis. Please choose the most appropriate diagnosis from the above list. Each diagnosis may be used once, more than once or not at all.

1. A 42-year-old woman presents to her GP with exertional dyspnoea associated with a dry cough and a bloody discharge from her nose. She has also noted swelling of her ankles and fingers. Subsequent investigations confirm acute renal failure and high titres of c-ANCA.

2. A 36-year-old man is admitted to hospital with a blood pressure of 210/130 mmHg and frank haematuria. Subsequent investigations reveal multiple renal aneurysms on renal angiography. The c-ANCA, the perinuclear ANCA (p-ANCA) and the extractable nuclear antigen (ENA) are all negative.

3. A 77-year-old woman presents to her GP with malaise and a severe bitemporal headache, associated with scalp tenderness. She denies any visual disturbance or other systemic upset. Her ESR is 110 mm/h.

4. A 22-year-old man presents to the Emergency Department with increasing wheeze and exertional dyspnoea. He has also noticed some ankle swelling. Investigations reveal: haemoglobin 11.2 g/dl, MCV 88 fl, WCC 13.6×10^9/l (eosinophils 11.2×10^9/l), platelets 221×10^9/l; Na$^+$ 132 mmol/l, K$^+$ 6.3 mmol/l, urea 17.9 mmol/l, and creatinine 472 μmol/l; the c-ANCA is negative.

5. A 27-year-old man presents to the Emergency Department with a severe rash over his shins, thighs and buttocks, associated with pain and swelling of his knees and ankles. His FBC, U&Es, autoantibody screen and urinalysis are unremarkable but the IgA levels are raised.

19. THEME: CHONDROCALCINOSIS

A   Acromegaly
B   Gout
C   Haemochromatosis
D   Hyperparathyroidism
E   Hypomagnesaemia
F   Hypothyroidism
G   Ochronosis
H   Pyrophosphate arthropathy
I   Trauma
J   Wilson's disease

The following patients have all presented with chondrocalcinosis. Please choose the most appropriate cause from the above list. Each option may be used once, more than once or not at all.

1. A 69-year-old man presents to his GP with a 4-day history of pain and swelling in his right knee. Examination confirms an acute arthritis of his knee but is otherwise unremarkable. Aspiration of the knee yeilds sterile fluid that contains crystals that are positively birefringent under polarised light.

2. A 37-year-old chronic alcohol abuser presents to her GP with weight loss, an 'unexpected sun tan' and pain in her lower limbs. Subsequent investigations reveal: glucose 17.8 mmol/l, total bilirubin 32 μmol/l, AST 324 IU/l, ALT 540 IU/l, alkaline phosphatase 123 IU/l, albumin 27 g/l, corrected Ca^{2+} 2.43 mmol/l, and PO_4^{3-} 0.78 mmol/l. Radiographs of her knees reveal 'intra-articular calcification'.

3. A 41-year-old woman presents to her GP with long-standing non-specific symptoms, including depression, lethargy and pain in her arms and legs. Routine investigations reveal widespread chondrocalcinosis and a corrected Ca^{2+} of 2.91 mmol/l.

4. A 52-year-old man presents to his GP with an acute exacerbation of his chronic arthritis. He is noted to have multiple exuding 'nodules' over his fingers and in his ear lobes. He improves with NSAID treatment.

5. A 71-year-old woman with vitiligo presents to her GP with increasing lethargy and a feeling of 'slowness'. She says that the arthritis in her hips and knees have also been 'playing up'. The GP notes that she has put on 14 kg in weight in the last year. Routine investigations reveal: haemoglobin 12.2 g/dl, MCV 104 fl, WCC 4.6 × 10⁹/l, platelets 321 × 10⁹/l; Na⁺ 125 mmol/l, K⁺ 4.3 mmol/l, urea 3.6 mmol/l, and creatinine 78 μmol/l.

20. THEME: RAISED ESR

A   Carcinomatosis
B   Miliary tuberculosis
C   Multiple myeloma
D   Polymyalgia rheumatica
E   Rheumatoid arthritis
F   Staphylococcal endocarditis
G   Temporal arteritis
H   Toxic shock syndrome
I   Ulcerative colitis
J   Wegener's granulomatosis

The following patients have all presented with an ESR of >100 mm/h. Please choose the most appropriate diagnosis from the above list. Each diagnosis may be used once, more than once or not at all.

1. A 74-year-old man presents to the Emergency Department with a 4-week history of increasing confusion and frank haemoptysis. Investigations reveal: Na$^+$ 121 mmol/l, K$^+$ 5.3 mmol/l, urea 23.6 mmol/l, creatinine 158 μmol/l; total bilirubin 43 μmol/l, ALT 299 IU/l, alkaline phosphatase 324 IU/l, albumin 31 g/l, corrected Ca^{2+} 3.06 mmol/l, and PO$_4^{3-}$ 0.78 mmol/l. The chest radiograph revealed 'multiple, large lesions throughout both lung fields'.

2. A 22-year-old woman is brought into the Emergency Department by ambulance having been found unconscious at home. On examination, she has a temperature of 39.5 °C, and is cold and clammy. The pulse 130 bpm, regular but thready; and the BP is 90/50 mmHg. A tampon is removed from her vagina by one of the Casualty nurses.

3. A 79-year-old man presents to the Emergency Department with a 3-week history of pains in his left humerus and right thigh, associated with increasing confusion. Investigations reveal: corrected Ca^{2+} 3.21 mmol/l, Bence Jones proteinuria, and a monoclonal IgG band on plasma electrophoresis.

4. A 64-year-old woman presents to her GP with aches and pains across the tops of her shoulders and thighs. She denies having any headaches or other systemic upset. Her routine blood tests are unremarkable other than an ESR of 102 mm/h.

5. A 23-year-old intravenous drug abuser presents in the Emergency Department with increasing shortness of breath associated with ankle oedema. Examination reveals him to be in gross cardiac failure with a loud early diastolic murmur at the left sternal edge.

21. THEME: AUTOANTIBODIES

A Anticardiolipin
B Anticentromere
C Anti-dsDNA
D Anti-Jo-1
E Anti-La
F Anti-RNP
G Anti-Ro
H Anti-Scl-70
I c-ANCA
J p-ANCA

The following patients have all presented with connective tissue disorders. Please choose the most characteristic autoantibody for each of their disorders from the above list. Each autoantibody may be used once, more than once or not at all.

1. A 23-year old woman presents to her GP with increasing malaise, which is associated with arthralgia and a rash over her upper cheeks. Routine investigations reveal a pancytopenia and mild renal impairment.

2. A 39-year old woman with long-standing pain and colour changes in her fingers in cold weather presents to her GP with multiple 'red spots' over her face and increasing dyspepsia. Recently she has been unable to open her mouth fully.

3. A 54-year old man presents to his GP with increasing pain and weakness of the upper limbs, associated with a rash around his eyes. Routine investigations reveal a creatine kinase of 22 500 IU/l and a large lesion in the right mid-zone on his chest radiograph.

4. A 36-year-old man presents to the Emergency Department with increasing shortness of breath on exertion and swelling of his ankles. He also admits to having a dry cough and a bloody nasal discharge. Routine investigations reveal: ESR 110 mm/h; Na^+ 128 mmol/l, K^+ 7.3 mmol/l, urea 53.6 mmol/l, creatinine 1158 μmol/l.

5. A 31-year-old woman presents to the Emergency Department with an acute, right-sided hemiparesis and facial palsy, associated with an expressive dysphasia. Of note, she has long-standing systemic lupus erythematosus (SLE) and had several miscarriages in her twenties.

22. THEME: RAYNAUD'S PHENOMENON

A   Cervical rib
B   Cold injury
C   Dermatomyositis
D   Ergot poisoning
E   Hypothyroidism
F   Lead poisoning
G   Sjögren's syndrome
H   SLE
I   Systemic sclerosis
J   Vibrating tools

The following patients have all presented with Raynaud's phenomenon. Please choose the most appropriate associated disorder from the above list. Each disorder may be used once, more than once or not at all.

1. A 35-year-old woman with a severe deforming arthropathy of her hands, elbows, hips and feet presents to her GP with symptoms suggestive of Raynaud's phenomenon. She also complains of a dry mouth and dry eyes. ☐

2. A 15-year-old schoolboy presents to his GP with pain and colour changes in the fingers of his right hand, which develop when exposed to the cold. He has also noted a buzzing around the right shoulder whilst lying in bed. ☐

3. A 49-year-old woman with vitiligo presents to her GP with increasing lethargy, weight gain and symptoms suggestive of Raynaud's phenomenon. On examination, she is noted to have early clubbing and a rash over her shins. ☐

4. A 32-year-old woman who has long-standing Raynaud's develops tightness and swelling of the fingers, associated with tightness around the mouth. Investigations reveal a mild normochromic anaemia and anticentromere antibodies. ☐

5. A 31-year-old woman visits her GP after developing an acute blistering rash. Of note, she had her first sunbed treatment the day before. On further questioning, she has had Raynaud's and aching joints and muscles for the past 3-4 months. Investigations reveal strongly positive ANA titres. ☐

23. THEME: BONE PROFILE ABNORMALITIES

A   Bony metastases
B   Chronic renal failure
C   DiGeorge's syndrome
D   Hyperparathyroidism
E   Multiple myeloma
F   Osteomalacia
G   Paget's bone disease
H   Pseudohypoparathyroidism
I   Parathyroid hormone-related polypeptide
J   Sarcoidosis

The following patients have all presented with an abnormal biochemical bone profile. Please choose the most appropriate diagnosis from the above list. Each diagnosis may be used once, more than once or not at all.

1. A 37-year-old man presents in the Emergency Department with a decreased level of consciousness and confusion. Examination reveals him to have a 'funny skin coloration', confusion but no focal neurological deficit, a pericardial rub and crepitations at the lung bases. Investigations reveal: haemoglobin 7.3 g/dl, MCV 91 fl, WCC 13.4 × 10^9/l, platelets 199 × 10^9/l; Na$^+$ 128 mmol/l, K$^+$ 8.1 mmol/l, urea 67.3 mmol/l, creatinine 911 μmol/l, corrected Ca^{2+} 1.67 mmol/l, PO$_4^{3-}$ 3.54 mmol/l, alkaline phosphatase 307 IU/l. ☐

2. A 79-year-old man presents with pain in his left hip and lower lumbar spine. Investigations reveal: Na$^+$ 134 mmol/l, K$^+$ 4.3 mmol/l, urea 5.4 mmol/l, creatinine 81 μmol/l; corrected Ca^{2+} 2.43 mmol/l, PO$_4^{3-}$ 0.74 mmol/l, alkaline phosphatase 421 IU/l; total bilirubin 12 μmol/l, AST 9 IU/l, ALT 14 IU/l, albumin 39 g/l. Radiographs of the pelvis show 'increased trabecular pattern with cortical thickening on the left side of the pelvis and femur'. ☐

3. A 49-year-old Bengali woman presents to her GP with non-specific aches and pains 'all over'. Examination is essentially normal. Investigations reveal: corrected Ca^{2+} 2.03 mmol/l, PO$_4^{3-}$ 0.31 mmol/l, alkaline phosphatase 511 IU/l; total bilirubin 9 μmol/l, AST 13 IU/l, ALT 11 IU/l, albumin 40 g/l. ☐

4. A 61-year-old lifelong smoker presents to his GP with gross weight loss and frank haemoptysis. Routine investigations reveal: Na$^+$ 127 mmol/l, K$^+$ 5.1 mmol/l, urea 7.6 mmol/l, creatinine 122 μmol/l; corrected Ca^{2+} 3.21 mmol/l, PO$_4^{3-}$ 0.61 mmol/l, alkaline phosphatase 342 IU/l; total bilirubin 42 μmol/l, AST 73 IU/l, ALT 64 IU/l, albumin 31 g/l. A chest radiograph shows a lesion in the right upper zone. A bone scan is unremarkable. ☐

5. A 71-year-old man is referred to Medical Outpatients with pains in his arms and legs, associated with lethargy and malaise. On examination, he has hepatosplenomegaly and is clinically anaemic, with areas of bruising and purpura. Investigations show: haemoglobin 6.7 g/dl, MCV 100 fl, WCC 21 × 10^9/l, platelets 23 × 10^9/l; Na$^+$ 130 mmol/l, K$^+$ 5.8 mmol/l, urea 21.9 mmol/l, creatinine 455 μmol/l; corrected Ca^{2+} 3.07 mmol/l, PO$_4^{3-}$ 0.41 mmol/l, alkaline phosphatase 601 IU/l; total bilirubin 62 μmol/l, AST 321 IU/l, ALT 564 IU/l, albumin 24 g/l; ESR 103 mm/h.

24. THEME: PROXIMAL MYOPATHY

A   Acromegaly
B   Alcoholic myopathy
C   Cushing's disease
D   Dermatomyositis
E   Diabetes mellitus
F   Duchenne's muscular dystrophy
G   Motor neurone disease
H   Osteomalacia
I   Polymyositis
J   Thyrotoxicosis

The following patients have all presented with proximal myopathy. Please choose the most appropriate diagnosis from the above list. Each diagnosis may be used once, more than once or not at all.

1. A 33-year-old woman presents to her GP with weight loss, sweats, weakness of the shoulders and palpitations. On examination, she is in fast atrial fibrillation and has lost 12 kg in weight over the past 8 months.

2. A 76-year-old man presents to his GP with generalised weakness of all four limbs, associated with weight loss and dysphagia and nasal regurgitation of food. On examination, he has a marked myopathy and a pseudobulbar palsy. Blood tests, including FBC, U&Es, LFTs, creatine kinase and thyroid function tests are all within normal limits.

3. A 42-year-old man presents to his GP with 'peripheral visual loss' and a feeling of tightness in his fingers and toes. The locum on duty notes that he has proximal myopathy, bitemporal hemianopia and hypertension, and refers him immediately to the hospital.

4. A 27-year-old woman presents to her GP with a 3-month history of increasing weight, polyuria and polydipsia and headaches. She also complains that her thighs and shoulders feel weak. On examination, she has gained 8 kg in weight and has marked abdominal striae, hypertension and a capillary blood glucose of 13.3 mmol/l.

5. A 41-year-old man presents to his GP with weakness and pain in his arms and legs. On examination, he is noted to have marked clubbing, Dupuytren's contracture, spider naevi and proximal myopathy. Routine investigations reveal: haemoglobin 12.9 g/dl, MCV 105 fl, WCC 3.9×10^9/l, platelets 45×10^9/l; Na^+ 129 mmol/l, K^+ 4.3 mmol/l, urea 2.4 mmol/l, creatinine 71 μmol/l; total bilirubin 32 μmol/l, AST 459 IU/l, ALT 614 IU/l, alkaline phosphatase 321 IU/l, albumin 21 g/l; and creatine kinase 21,000 IU/l.

Endocrine, Breast, Dermatology

1. THEME: HYPOTHALAMIC AND PITUITARY DISEASE

A   Acromegaly
B   Cranial diabetes insipidus
C   Craniopharyngioma
D   Cushing's syndrome
E   Kallmann's syndrome
F   Lactotroph pituitary macroadenoma
G   Lactotroph pituitary microadenoma
H   Nelson's syndrome
I   Nephrogenic diabetes insipidus
J   Sheehan's syndrome

The patients below have all presented with symptoms suggestive of hypothalamic or pituitary disease. Choose the most appropriate diagnosis from the above list. Each diagnosis may be used once, more than once or not at all.

1. A 27-year-old woman presents to her GP with lethargy, fatigue, weight gain, impaired short-term memory and secondary amenorrhoea, which has persisted since the delivery of her son 1 year ago. She was unable to breastfeed her baby because her milk dried up over 2 days. The labour was complicated by a 3-litre post-partum haemorrhage.

2. A 58-year-old man who underwent bilateral adrenalectomy 30 years ago for the treatment of Cushing's disease, and who has noticed increasing pigmentation of his skin over the past 5 years, presents to his GP with headache and double vision. The GP finds a right sixth cranial nerve palsy. Urgent magnetic resonance imaging (MRI) demonstrates a pituitary tumour that is invading the right cavernous sinus.

3. A 24-year-old woman who recently suffered a subarachnoid haemorrhage develops polyuria, with a urine output of 400 ml/h, in the hours following surgery to clip an aneurysm of the anterior communicating artery.

4. A 41-year-old man presents to his GP with visual loss after a near miss with a bus. The GP finds a bitemporal hemianopia and elicits a history of headache, lethargy, loss of libido and impotence. Thyroid function tests are normal but the 9 am cortisol is below the normal range and the prolactin is 97 000 mU/l.

5. A 16-year-old girl presents to Endocrinology Out-patients with primary amenorrhoea and delayed puberty. She has been anosmic since birth. Baseline investigations establish that she has normal pituitary function with the exception of a low levels of luteinising hormone, follicle-stimulating hormone and oestradiol.

2. THEME: DISORDERS OF THE HYPOTHALAMO-PITUITARY-ADRENAL AXIS

A   Addison's disease
B   Adrenal adenoma
C   Adrenal carcinoma
D   Adrenal tuberculosis
E   Cushing's disease
F   Ectopic adrenocorticotrophic hormone (ACTH) secretion
G   Iatrogenic Addison's syndrome
H   Iatrogenic Cushing's syndrome
I   Pseudo-Cushing's syndrome
J   Waterhouse–Friderichsen syndrome

The patients below have all presented with disorders associated with the steroid axis. Choose the most appropriate diagnosis from the above list. Each diagnosis may be used once, more than once or not at all.

1. A 51-year-old woman on regular vitamin B_{12} replacement for pernicious anaemia presents to her GP with weight loss, fatigue and depression. The GP notes postural hypotension, buccal pigmentation and widespread patchy vitiligo. The FBC is normal but the U&Es reveal: Na^+ 135 mmol/l, K^+ 5.7 mmol/l, urea 8.1 mmol/l and creatinine 69 μmol/l.

2. A 29-year-old woman presents to Endocrinology Out-patients with a 4-month history of hirsutism, secondary amenorrhoea and weight gain. Examination reveals clitoromegaly, greasy skin, acne, male-pattern hair growth and centripetal obesity. The 9 am serum cortisol is grossly elevated, and ACTH is undetectable.

3. A 61-year-old man presents to Endocrinology Out-patients with a 3-month history of weight loss, loss of libido and fatigue. Examination reveals a plethoric face, thin skin, easy bruising, hyperpigmentation, hypertension and glycosuria. The serum cortisol and plasma ACTH levels are elevated and fail to suppress on a high-dose dexamethasone suppression test. MRI pituitary is normal. A CT scan of the abdomen shows bilateral adrenal nodular hyperplasia.

4. A 20-year-old man presents to his GP with a 2-year history of weight gain, weakness and depression. Examination reveals a plethoric, moon-shaped face, thin skin, a buffalo hump, centripetal obesity and proximal myopathy. Serum cortisol and plasma ACTH levels, which are both high, suppress after high-dose, but not after low-dose dexamethasone suppression.

5. A 53-year-old man presents to his GP with a long history of weight gain, fatigue and depression. Examination reveals a plethoric, moon-shaped face, thin skin, a buffalo hump, centripetal obesity, red abdominal striae, proximal myopathy and depression. The serum cortisol is elevated and fails to suppress on low-dose dexamethasone suppression. A FBC shows macrocytosis. MRI pituitary is normal. Abdominal CT shows normal adrenals and hepatomegaly.

3. THEME: THYROID DISEASE

A Anaplastic carcinoma
B Follicular carcinoma
C Graves' disease
D Hashimoto's thyroiditis
E Medullary thyroid carcinoma
F Multinodular goitre
G Papillary carcinoma
H Simple colloid goitre
I Thyroglossal cyst
J Thyroid adenoma

The patients below have all presented with conditions of the thyroid. Please select the most appropriate diagnosis from the above list. Each diagnosis may be used once, more than once or not at all.

1. A 30-year-old woman presents with an enlarging painless lump to the left of the midline in the lower third of the neck. The lump is soft, non-tender and moves on swallowing. The thyroid function tests show: free thyroxine (fT4) 40 pmol/l, thyroid-stimulating hormone (TSH) not detectable.

2. A 70-year-old woman presents with a 2-month history of swelling in the neck associated with an aching pain and, more recently, hoarseness and some difficulty in breathing. Examination reveals a large hard mass in the region of the left thyroid lobe with an irregular surface and an indistinct edge. The patient has stridor and left cervical lymphadenopathy and indirect laryngoscopy reveals paralysis of the left cord. The thyroid function tests are normal.

3. A 22-year-old woman presents with a 6 month history of progressive weight loss despite having a ravenous appetite. She also comments that she always feels warm and finds hot weather unpleasant. Her partner says that he is finding it increasingly difficult to live with her irritability. On examination, there is very slight, smooth enlargement of the whole gland and a bruit is audible. The thyroid function tests show: fT_4 250 pmol/l, TSH not detectable.

4. A 26-year-old pregnant woman presents with a 3-month history of a slowly growing, asymptomatic swelling in the neck. On examination, the gland feels smoothly enlarged but the architecture is preserved. Thyroid function tests show: fT_4 18 pmol/l, TSH 5.4 mU/l.

5. A 28-year-old man presents with headaches to his GP, who finds that he is profoundly hypertensive. He is referred to hospital, where specialist investigations reveal a normal FBC, normal U&Es, corrected Ca^{2+} 2.90 mmol/l, PO_4^{3-} 0.75 mmol/l, immunoreactive parathyroid hormone (PTH) 150 pg/ml, fT_4 18 pmol/l, TSH 0.35 mU/l, and raised 24-hour urinary catecholamines. The thyroid gland appears normal on examination. Abdominal CT revealed an adrenal mass.

4. THEME: HYPERGLYCAEMIA

A   Acromegaly
B   Bendroflumethiazide
C   Chronic pancreatitis
D   Cushing's disease
E   Gestational diabetes
F   Glucagonoma
G   Haemochromatosis
H   Prednisolone
I   Thyrotoxicosis
J   Type 1 diabetes mellitus

The patients below all have hyperglycaemia. Choose the most likely diagnosis from the above list. Each diagnosis may be used once, more than once or not at all.

1. A 54-year-old actor presents to his GP with polyuria, polydipsia and a 2-year history of weight loss, recurrent abdominal discomfort and pale, foul-smelling stools.

2. A 36-year-old woman presents to her GP with secondary amenorrhoea and a negative pregnancy test. On further questioning she admits to nocturia, polyuria, lethargy, excessive sweating, headache and galactorrhoea. Last year she underwent bilateral carpal tunnel decompression and had to have her wedding ring enlarged.

3. A 17-year-old boy presents to his GP with a 3-week history of lethargy, weakness, polyuria, polydipsia and weight loss.

4. A 46-year-old man presents to his GP with polyuria and polydipsia and 1-year history of joint aches and pains, upper abdominal discomfort, fatigue and impotence. On examination, he appears suntanned and there is smooth, firm hepatomegaly.

5. A previously healthy 31-year-old man presents to his GP with polyuria and polydipsia and a 2-year history of weight gain, fatigue, weakness, easy bruising, loss of libido and depression.

5. THEME: COMPLICATIONS OF DIABETES

A Amyotrophy
B Autonomic neuropathy
C Cerebrovascular disease
D Diabetic nephropathy
E Hypertriglyceridaemia
F Ischaemic heart disease
G Mononeuritis multiplex
H Peripheral sensory neuropathy
I Recurrent urinary tract infection
J Retinopathy

The patients below have all presented with complications of their diabetes. Choose the most appropriate diagnosis from the above list. Each complication may be used once, more than once or not at all.

1. A 31-year-old man with type 1 diabetes mellitus presents to his GP with balance problems, which manifest only in the dark. Fundoscopy and visual acuity are normal but there is loss of proprioception bilaterally in the toes and ankles, and a small painless ulcer is evident beneath the left first metatarsal head.

2. A 77-year-old man with type 2 diabetes mellitus presents to his GP with a 2-month history of pain in the right upper leg. On examination, the right quadriceps is wasted and very tender, with an absent reflex.

3. A 62-year-old woman with type 2 diabetes mellitus presents to the Diabetes Clinic with gradual onset of weakness of the left hand and forearm. On examination, there is a flaccid paresis of the wrist extensors and flexors, the muscles of the thenar and hypothenar eminences and the small muscles of the hand. Sensation is intact.

4. A 38-year-old man with type 1 diabetes mellitus and hypertension is found to have proteinuria on dipstick testing. Blood tests show a normal urea and creatinine and a normocytic normochromic anaemia.

5. A 78-year-old woman with type 2 diabetes mellitus presents to the Emergency Department after a fall. She has fallen frequently over the past 6 months, always on rising from a chair. Her BP is 146/72 mmHg lying and 98/50 mmHg standing.

6. THEME: DIABETIC EYE DISEASE

A Background retinopathy
B Central retinal artery occlusion
C Central retinal vein occlusion
D Cortical blindness
E Maculopathy
F Optic atrophy
G Pre-proliferative retinopathy
H Proliferative retinopathy
I Snowflake cataracts
J Vitreous haemorrhage

The patients below have presented with eye disease related to their diabetes mellitus. Choose the most appropriate diagnosis from the above list. Each diagnosis may be used once, more than once or not at all.

1. Dilated fundoscopy in a 48-year-old man with type 2 diabetes mellitus demonstrates widespread microaneurysms, blot haemorrhages and hard exudates, with macular sparing.

2. A 53-year-old man presents to his GP with sudden, total loss of vision in the right eye. Fundoscopy reveals loss of the red reflex with a grey haze obscuring the retina.

3. Dilated fundoscopy in a 34-year-old man with type 1 diabetes mellitus reveals microaneurysms, blot haemorrhages, hard exudates, cotton-wool spots and new vessels.

4. A 62-year-old woman presents to the Emergency Department having suffered sudden, profound visual loss in the right eye. On examination, visual acuity on the right is limited to perception of light only. The fundus is pale with a cherry-red spot at the macula.

5. A 49-year-old woman presents to the Emergency Department with sudden, profound visual loss in the right eye. Fundoscopy reveals a grossly swollen optic disc with cotton-wool spots and haemorrhages throughout the retina.

7. THEME: DRUG COMPLICATIONS IN PATIENTS WITH DIABETES

A   Acarbose
B   Amlodipine
C   Bendroflumethiazide
D   Chlorpropamide
E   Glibenclamide
F   Human insulin
G   Metformin
H   Propranolol
I   Rosiglitazone

The diabetic patients below have all presented with side-effects of their medication. Choose the most appropriate cause from the list above. Each drug may be used once, more than once or not at all.

1. A 58-year-old man with type 2 diabetes mellitus begins to suffer from disabling flatulence shortly after a new drug is added to his medications.

2. A 45-year-old man with type 1 diabetes mellitus notices that he has become less aware of impending hypoglycaemia since the introduction of an antihypertensive.

3. A 49-year-old woman with type 2 diabetes mellitus whose medication has recently been changed begins to suffer an unpleasant facial flushing sensation after drinking alcohol.

4. A 63-year-old woman with insulin-controlled type 2 diabetes mellitus notices that her insulin requirement increases after starting treatment with an antihypertensive.

5. A 70 year-old man with type 2 diabetes mellitus and staphylococcal septicaemia arising from an infected right foot becomes increasingly dyspnoeic. Arterial blood gases show: pH 7.24, PCO_2 3.0 kPa, PO_2 14.1 kPa, HCO_3^- 15 mmol/l, base excess −12 mmol/l.

8. THEME: ADVERSE EFFECTS OF ENDOCRINE DRUGS

A   Alendronate
B   Calcitonin
C   Carbimazole
D   Chlorpropamide
E   Clomifene
F   Metformin
G   Mixtard® insulin
H   Octreotide
I   Prednisolone
J   Thyroxine

The patients below have all presented with adverse effects of their endocrine treatments. Choose the most appropriate drug from the above list. Each drug may be used once, more than once or not at all.

1. A 64-year-old woman presents to her GP with a sore throat. The FBC shows: haemoglobin 11.4 g/dl, WCC 1.9×10^9/l, platelets 154×10^9/l, no neutrophils, lymphocytes 1.9×10^9/l.

2. A 47-year-old man presents to the Emergency Department with right upper quadrant abdominal pain and jaundice. Ultrasound scan shows biliary dilatation and multiple gallstones. A large gallstone is retrieved from the common bile duct during ERCP.

3. A 72-year-old man has an abnormality picked up on routine blood testing. His investigations show: Na$^+$ 129 mmol/l, K$^+$ 4.1 mmol/l, Cl$^-$ 100 mmol/l, HCO$_3^-$ 26 mmol/l, urea 6.2 mmol/l, creatinine 91 μmol/l.

4. A 27-year-old woman presents to the Emergency Department with acute severe lower abdominal pain. Ultrasound examination shows massive cystic enlargement of both ovaries and ascites.

5. A 55-year-old woman presents to her GP with retrosternal pain. ECG and chest radiography are normal but gastroscopy reveals severe oesophageal erosions and ulceration.

9. THEME: LUMPS IN THE BREAST

A   Acute pyogenic mastitis
B   Cyst
C   Duct ectasia
D   Fat necrosis
E   Fibroadenoma
F   Fibrocystic change
G   Intraduct papilloma
H   Invasive ductal carcinoma
I   Lipoma
J   Radial scar

For each of the patients below, select the most likely cause of a lump in the breast from the above list. Each option may be used once, more than once or not at all.

B/C

1. A 34 year old woman presents with an ill-defined lump in the left breast that enlarges and becomes tender in the second half of the menstrual cycle. ☐

2. A 65-year-old woman presents with a hard lump in the upper outer quadrant of the left breast. On examination, enlarged ipsilateral axillary nodes are also present. Mammography shows a 3-cm stellate mass with microcalcification. H

3. A 56-year-old woman presents with discharge of thick, creamy fluid from the right nipple. On examination, there is a poorly defined subareolar mass. Ultrasound of the breast shows dilated subareolar ducts. Cytological examination of the discharge fluid shows macrophages and debris but no epithelial cells. ABC C

4. A 22-year-old woman presents with a 3-cm mobile lump that is solid and has well-defined margins on ultrasound. Fine needle aspiration cytology (FNAC) shows benign cells. E

5. A 31-year-old woman presents with an ill-defined tender mass in the upper outer quadrant of the left breast 2 weeks after giving birth. On examination, the affected segment is diffusely red and hot. FNAC of the mass shows neutrophils and inflammatory debris but no malignant cells. A

10. THEME: GENERAL RASHES

A   Acanthosis nigricans
B   Dermatitis herpetiformis
C   Erythema ab igne
D   Erythema multiforme
E   Erythema nodosum
F   Herpes zoster
G   Lupus vulgaris
H   Necrobiosis lipoidica
I   Pyoderma gangrenosum
J   Rosacea

The patients below have all presented with rashes. Please choose the most appropriate diagnosis from the above list. Each diagnosis may be used once, more than once or not at all.

1. An 89-year-old woman is brought to the Emergency Department having been found unconscious at home by a neighbour. On examination, she is pyrexial and very confused and is noted to have coarse crackles at the right lung base. Over the anterolateral aspects of her lower legs there is a reticular, pigmented rash.

2. A 39-year-old woman presents to her GP with an erythematous, papular rash affecting her cheeks, forehead and chin. Also of note, she has suffered with 'flushing' when hot or stressed for several years.

3. A 41-year-old woman with known diabetes mellitus presents to her GP with a thickened, pigmented, waxy-looking rash over the anterior aspect of her left shin.

4. A 36-year-old Bengali man presents to his GP with a 3-month history of weight loss, night sweats and a productive cough. He has also noted a scaly, plaque-like rash over the extensor surface of his left elbow.

5. An 18-year-old student presents to her GP with a 6-week history of an extremely pruritic rash. On examination, she is well but has a diffuse, symmetrical rash, principally over the extensor surfaces of her limbs. The rash is heavily excoriated and erythematous and is both papular and vesicular. Subsequent skin biopsy from an unaffected area shows subepidermal IgA deposition.

11. THEME: BLISTERING RASHES

A Dermatitis herpetiformis
B Epidermolysis bullosa
C Herpes simplex virus
D Herpes zoster virus
E Insect bites
F Pemphigoid
G Pemphigus
H *Staphylococcus*
I Stevens–Johnson syndrome
J Variegate porphyria

The patients below have all presented with blistering rashes. Please choose the most appropriate diagnosis from the above list. Each diagnosis may be used once, more than once or not at all.

1. A 33-year-old man presents to the Emergency Department with a 2-week history of worsening fevers, dyspnoea and a cough productive of greenish sputum. In the last 24 hours he has developed a severe blistering rash affecting all areas of his skin and oral mucosa, associated with 'sticky, painful eyes'.

2. A 21-year-old woman presents in the Emergency Department with a blistering rash over her knees, elbows and buttocks. In the last 3 months she has lost 4-5 kg in weight and has had 'diarrhoea'. Investigations reveal a macrocytic anaemia and highly positive antiendomysial antibody titres.

3. An 83-year-old woman living in a nursing home is seen by her GP. She is becoming increasingly confused and has a severe blistering rash over her abdomen. Her urinalysis shows: blood + +, protein +++, nitrites ++. The rash over the abdomen is confined to a band radiating from her left loin to the umbilicus.

4. An 86-year-old man presents in the Emergency Department with tense blisters over his limbs and chest. The blisters vary in size from a few millimetres to a few centimetres in diameter. There are no lesions over the genitalia, buccal mucosa or eyes.

5. A 67-year-old woman presents in the Emergency Department with a blistering rash. On examination, she is unwell and has multiple blisters of varying size, many of which have become sloughy and de-roofed. The underlying skin is erythematous and 'raw'. There are denuded areas around the eyes and several lesions affecting the buccal mucosa.

12. THEME: DERMATITIS

A   Asteatotic eczema
B   Atopic eczema
C   Contact dermatitis
D   Eczema herpeticum
E   Exfoliative dermatitis
F   Nummular dermatitis
G   Pityriasis alba
H   Seborrhoeic dermatitis

The patients below have all presented with dermatitis. Please choose the most appropriate diagnosis from the above list. Each diagnosis may be used once, more than once or not at all.

1. An 8-year-old schoolboy with known hay fever presents to his GP with an erythematous, dry, scaling rash affecting his hands, the flexor surfaces of his upper and lower limbs, and his face. There is marked lichenification and there are excoriated areas.

2. A 7-year-old Asian girl presents to her GP with a mild eczematous rash, principally over her lower limbs. There are areas of depigmentation around her knees.

3. An 87-year-old woman is admitted to hospital with confusion following a fall. Three days later she develops an eczematous, 'crazy paving-'like rash over the anterior aspects of her legs.

4. A 21-year-old trainee hairdresser presents to his GP with a 3-week history of a 'raw', erythematous rash over both hands.

5. A 14-year-old schoolboy presents to his GP with an itchy rash affecting his upper and lower limbs. On examination, he has symmetrically distributed, discrete, round patches of eczema.

13. THEME: PRURITUS

A   Candidiasis
B   Eczema
C   Hypothyroidism
D   Insect bites
E   Iron deficiency
F   Jaundice
G   Lymphoma
H   Psoriasis
I   Scabies
J   Uraemia

The patients below have all presented with pruritus. Please choose the most appropriate diagnosis from the above list. Each diagnosis may be used once, more than once or not at all.

1. A 49-year-old 'down and out' presents in the Emergency Department after a fall. On examination, he has a swollen right ankle due to a soft-tissue injury. He is unkempt and is distressed by an extremely itchy rash over both hands. The dorsum of both hands is heavily excoriated and there are 'papules' between the finger webs.

2. A 39-year-old woman presents to her GP with lethargy, severe pruritus and night sweats. Examination reveals generalised lymphadenopathy, weight loss and hepatosplenomegaly.

3. A 26-year-old woman presents to her GP with a dry, pruritic, scaling rash affecting the extensor surfaces of her elbows and knees, as well as her scalp. Her nails are heavily pitted and ridged.

4. An 81-year-old man presents to the Emergency Department with a 6-month history of increasing confusion, associated with weight loss and occasional dysphagia. On examination, he has pruritus marks over his anterior abdomen, a Virchow's node and a palpable epigastric mass.

5. A 42-year-old man with known ischaemic heart disease and type 2 diabetes mellitus is started on an ACE inhibitor by his GP. Six weeks later he presents in the Emergency Department with nausea and vomiting, pruritus and increasing confusion.

14. THEME: CHANGES IN PIGMENTATION

A   Acanthosis nigricans
B   Addison's disease
C   Amiodarone therapy
D   Ectopic ACTH secretion
E   Gold therapy
F   Haemochromatosis
G   Leprosy
H   Pernicious anaemia
I   Pityriasis versicolor
J   Vitiligo

The patients below have all presented with changes in skin pigmentation. Please choose the most appropriate diagnosis from the above list. Each diagnosis may be used once, more than once or not at all.

1. A 49-year-old smoker presents to his GP with extreme lethargy and weakness, haemoptysis and an 'unexpected suntan'. Initial investigations reveal: haemoglobin 10.9 g/dl, MCV 85.2 fl, WCC 13.6×10^9/l, platelets 245×10^9/l; Na$^+$ 136 mmol/l, K$^+$ 2.3 mmol/l, urea 4.4 mmol/l, creatinine 91 μmol/l.

2. A 37-year-old woman presents to her GP a few days after returning from her summer holiday. Her husband has noted areas of depigmentation interspersed with her suntan, particularly over her back. The lesions improve with itraconazole cream.

3. A 29-year-old woman with known hypothyroidism presents to her GP with menorrhagia. On examination, she is clinically well but obviously anaemic. Areas of depigmentation over the dorsum of both hands are noticed as an incidental finding.

4. A 28-year-old woman presents to her GP with lethargy and weakness. On examination, she is extremely thin and pale, has marked pigmentation of her palmar creases, and an old appendix scar. Initial investigations reveal: BP 100/70 mmHg sitting, 80/60 mmHg standing, capillary blood glucose 3.8 mmol/l.

5. A 31-year-old, obese, diabetic man is seen in the Diabetic Clinic for his 6-monthly check-up. The ST2 doctor notes that he has a dark, velvety lesion covering the nape of his neck and in both axillae.

15. THEME: NAIL DISORDERS

A   Clubbing
B   Koilonychia
C   Leuconychia
D   Onychogryphosis
E   Onycholysis
F   Paronychia
G   Pitting
H   Ridging
I   Splinter haemorrhages
J   Yellow nails

The patients below have all presented with abnormalities of their nails. Please choose the most appropriate diagnosis from the above list. There may be more than one correct choice for each scenario, and the options may be used more than once.

1. A 33-year-old man with a previous history of rheumatic fever presents to his GP with a 4-month history of increasing exertional dyspnoea and lethargy. On examination, he has abnormal nails, tender nodules in the pulp of his fingers and a loud pansystolic murmur at the apex. He is also noted to have basal crepitations and ankle oedema.

2. A 29-year-old woman presents to her GP with weight loss, 'irritability' and heat intolerance. On examination, she has abnormal nails and a fine tremor and has a resting tachycardia.

3. A 42-year-old chronic alcohol abuser presents to his GP with jaundice. On examination, he has abnormal nails, palmar erythema and pruritus marks. He is jaundiced and has ascites and hepatosplenomegaly.

4. An 82-year-old man with worsening visual impairment and mobility is referred to a geriatric day hospital for further investigation. While helping him to get undressed, the nurse notices that his toenails are extremely 'overgrown and dystrophic'.

5. A 58-year-old woman with a previous history of tuberculosis presents to her GP with an 8-month history of exertional dyspnoea and a cough productive of copious amounts of green sputum. A chest radiograph shows: 'evidence of old tuberculosis infection with marked basal tramlines and air trapping, particularly on the left'.

16. THEME: ERYTHEMA NODOSUM

A   Acute lymphoblastic leukaemia
B   Epstein–Barr virus
C   Histoplasmosis
D   Hodgkin's disease
E   Inflammatory bowel disease
F   Oral contraceptive pill
G   Pregnancy
H   Sarcoidosis
I   *Streptococcus*
J   Tuberculosis

The patients below have all presented with erythema nodosum. Please choose the most appropriate underlying cause from the above list. Each option may be used once, more than once or not at all.

1. A 34-year-old man presents to his GP with worsening exertional dyspnoea, lethargy and a painful rash over the shins. His chest radiograph shows bilateral hilar lymphadenopathy with no other abnormalities. He has a raised serum ACE and his serum corrected Ca^{2+} is 2.76 mmol/l.

2. A 41-year-old alcohol abuser presents to the Emergency Department with a 2-month history of weight loss, night sweats and purulent yellow sputum. On examination, he has cervical lymphadenopathy, coarse crackles in the right upper and mid-zones and a rash over the shins.

3. A 26-year-old woman with a previous history of severe and prolonged Epstein–Barr infection presents to her GP with a 3-week history of worsening swelling under both arms and in the neck, associated with night sweats. On examination she is noted to be thin, and she has generalised lymphadenopathy and erythema nodosum. Routine investigations reveal: haemoglobin 7.9 g/dl, MCV 89 fl, WCC 45.2 × 10⁹/l (lymphocytes 41.2 × 10⁹/l), platelets 301 × 10⁹/l; ESR 78 mm/h.

4. A 16-year-old schoolgirl is seen by her GP for fever, swollen glands in the neck, a sore throat and an erythematous, painful rash over the shins. A blood film that day confirms a positive monospot test.

5. An 85-year-old man presents in the Emergency Department after a collapse. On examination, he is pyrexial, he has bronchial breathing and coarse crackles in the left upper and mid-zones and he has an erythematous rash over his shins. A chest radiograph shows a left upper lobe pneumonia and subsequent sputum microscopy reveals Gram-positive cocci.

17. THEME: ERYTHEMA MULTIFORME

A Bronchial carcinoma
B Herpes simplex virus
C Histoplasmosis
D *Mycoplasma*
E Orf virus
F Rheumatoid arthritis
G *Streptococcus*
H SLE
I Tuberculosis
J Ulcerative colitis

The patients below have all presented with erythema multiforme. Please choose the most appropriate underlying cause from the above list. Each cause may be used once, more than once or not at all.

1. A 12-year-old schoolboy is admitted to hospital with a severe headache and a depressed level of consciousness. His mother says he has had a sore throat for 2-3 days. His ASOT is highly positive and CSF obtained by lumbar puncture shows a raised protein concentration and reduced glucose. Ten days later he develops a severe blistering rash affecting his limbs and oral mucosa.

2. A 39-year-old man presents to his GP with a blistering rash, dry cough and fever. He is subsequently admitted to hospital, where investigations reveal: haemoglobin 13.2 g/dl, MCV 85.2 fl, WCC 12.6 × 10⁹/l, platelets 265 × 10⁹/l; Na⁺ 126 mmol/l, K⁺ 5.3 mmol/l, urea 5.4 mmol/l, creatinine 71 μmol/l; total bilirubin 34 μmol/l, albumin 38 g/l, AST 45 IU/l, alkaline phosphatase 126 IU/l. His chest radiograph shows: 'patchy shadowing in the left and right lung fields'.

3. A 22-year-old man presents to his GP with a blistering rash affecting his limbs, back, chest, abdomen and oral mucosa. Over the past 3 months he has suffered weight loss and bloody diarrhoea.

4. A 24-year-old woman presents to her GP with a rash over her cheeks, arthritis, swollen ankles and an erythema multiforme-like rash. Initial investigations reveal: Na⁺ 129 mmol/l, K⁺ 6.3 mmol/l, urea 35.4 mmol/l, creatinine 671 μmol/l; ESR 91 mm/h, rheumatoid factor negative, dsDNA antibodies highly positive.

5. A 31-year-old woman presents to her GP with a florid blistering rash over her upper and lower limbs, associated with a healing, 'scabbing' lesion on the right side of her upper lip.

18. THEME: PYODERMA GANGRENOSUM

A   Acute lymphoblastic leukaemia
B   Ankylosing spondylitis
C   Crohn's disease
D   Multiple myeloma
E   Myelofibrosis
F   Primary thrombocythaemia
G   Rheumatoid arthritis
H   Ulcerative colitis
I   Waldenström's macroglobulinaemia
J   Wegener's granulomatosis

The patients below have all presented with pyoderma gangrenosum. Please choose the most appropriate diagnosis from the above list. Each diagnosis may be used once, more than once or not at all.

1. A 26-year-old man presents to his GP with an ulcerating lesion over the dorsum of his left hand, a vasculitic rash, and haemoptysis. Subsequent investigations reveal: haemoglobin 10.9 g/dl, MCV 88 fl, WCC 14.9 × 10⁹/l, platelets 200 × 10⁹/l; Na⁺ 130 mmol/l, K⁺ 6.3 mmol/l, urea 19.9 mmol/l, creatinine 383 μmol/l; ESR 112 mm/h, rheumatoid factor and dsDNA antibodies both negative, c-ANCA highly positive.

2. A 61-year-old woman presents to her GP with an ulcerating lesion over the shin of her left leg. On further questioning, she gives a 3-month history of lethargy and easy bruising. On examination she is clinically anaemic, with multiple bruises and massive splenomegaly. Subsequent investigations reveal: haemoglobin 6.1 g/dl, MCV 83 fl, WCC 74.9 × 10⁹/l, platelets 13 × 10⁹/l; Philadelphia chromosome negative. Bone marrow aspiration was unsuccessful.

3. A 72-year-old man presents to his GP with lethargy and exertional dyspnoea. On examination, he is clinically anaemic and heavily bruised but has no palpable lymphadenopathy or hepatosplenomegaly. Investigations reveal: haemoglobin 5.8 g/dl, MCV 94 fl, WCC 2.2 × 10⁹/l, platelets 21 × 10⁹/l; ESR 110 mm/h; corrected Ca²⁺ 2.32 mmol/l. Plasma electrophoresis showed IgM paraproteinaemia. No lytic lesions were seen on a chest radiograph.

4. A 19-year-old man presents to his GP with low back and buttock pain, now associated with an ulcerating lesion on his right shin. Radiographs of the pelvis and lumbar spine show 'erosions of the sacroiliac joints'.

5. A 29-year-old man with known episodic bloody diarrhoea presents to his GP with a 2-week history of an ulcerating lesion over the shin of his right leg. Previous colonic biopsies have shown 'superficial ulceration with reduced numbers of goblet cells and multiple crypt abscesses'.

CHAPTER **5**

Paediatrics

Paediatrics

1. THEME: INTERVENTIONS FOR ABNORMAL HEART RHYTHM

A   Intravenous adenosine
B   Intravenous adrenaline/epinephrine
C   Intravenous amiodarone
D   Asynchronous shock
E   Intravenous atropine
F   Bag-valve-mask ventilation
G   Carotid sinus massage
H   Intravenous lidocaine
I   No intervention from this list
J   Synchronous shock

The following patients all have abnormal heart rates. Please select the most useful first intervention from the above list. Each option may be used once, more than once or not at all.

1. A newborn infant is born by elective Caesarian. He is pink, well perfused and breathing normally. His oxygen saturation is 98% and his heart rate 75 bpm.

2. A male infant is delivered by forceps after a prolonged labour. He is pale, apnoeic and has a heart rate of 20 bpm.

3. An 8-year-old known diabetic is admitted in severe ketoacidosis. His BP is 60/30 mmHg and his heart rate is 195 bpm.

4. A 9-month-old baby who has had surgery for complex congenital cyanotic cardiac disease collapses on the ward 2 days post-operatively. There is no palpable pulse and the ECG shows ventricular tachycardia at 260 bpm.

5. A 6-month-old baby girl is brought into the Emergency Department with poor feeding and 'not being herself'. Examination is normal except for a heart rate of 230 bpm. Vagal manoeuvres are tried but do not help.

2. THEME: CAUSES OF HYPERTENSION

A Coarctation of the aorta
B Congenital adrenal hyperplasia
C Essential hypertension
D Glomerulonephritis
E Haemolytic-uraemic syndrome
F Iatrogenic
G ~~Neuroblastoma~~ Nephroblastoma
H Patent ductus arteriosus
I Phaeochromocytoma
J Renal artery stenosis

The following children have been found to have a high blood pressure. Please select the most likely cause from the list of conditions above. All measurements are from the right arm. Each diagnosis may be used once, more than once or not at all.

1. An 8-year-old is undergoing remission induction therapy for leukaemia. At diagnosis he was found to have a short, soft sytolic murmur audible over the upper left sternal edge but, other than his pallor, lymphadenopathy and petechial haemorrhages, is normal on examination. His BP is 130/90 mmHg.

2. A 2-year-old girl is being seen because of her small stature and possible dysmorphism. She has a systolic murmur in the subclavicular region that radiates to the back, grade 2/6. Her BP is 130/90 mmHg.

3. After several days of bloody diarrhoea, a 2-year-old girl is found to have developed pallor and purpura. Her BP is 130/80 mmHg. Blood tests show anaemia and a raised creatinine level.

4. A 16-year-old girl is seen in the Endocrine Clinic for further investigation of her delayed puberty. Urine catecholamines are normal, and there are no cells in the urine. She has a BP of 140/90 mmHg.

5. A 4-year-old presents with pallor and abdominal distension. Examination reveals a BP of 120/80 mmHg and a 5-cm mass to the left of the umbilicus.

3. THEME: CHOICE OF ANTIBIOTIC

A Intraveous benzylpenicillin and gentamicin
B Intravenous cefotaxime
C Intravenous co-amoxiclav (Augmentin®)
D Intravenous vancomycin
E No intervention from this list
F Oral Amoxil®
G Oral azithromycin
H Oral penicillin V
I Oral trimethoprim
J Oral vancomycin

The following children have an infection. Please select the antibiotic most likely to be beneficial for the child from the options above. Each antibiotic may be used once, more than once or not at all.

1. A 7-year-old with severe spastic quadraplegia develops a cough, respiratory distress and is desaturated in air.

2. A 5-year-old has recovered from meningococcal septicaemia. On day 9 of treatment she develops severe watery diarrhoea with abdominal pain and a fever. Stool culture is positive for *Clostridium difficile* toxin.

3. A 3-year-old boy with a Hickman line, sited for treatment of his neuroblastoma, has developed a fever. Cultures have shown a coagulase-negative staphylococcus.

4. A pre-term infant develops respiratory distress 2 hours after birth. The chest radiograph shows generalised air bronchograms and a ground-glass appearance.

5. A 4-year-old boy has a cough and a temperature of 37.9 °C. Examination reveals a reddened throat and inflammation of both tympanic membranes.

4. THEME: CAUSES OF LYMPHADENOPATHY

A   Acute lymphoblastic leukaemia
B   Acute myeloid leukaemia
C   Cat scratch disease
D   Epstein–Barr viral infection
E   HIV infection
F   Kawasaki's disease
G   Lymphoma
H   Reaction to local infection
I   Rubella
J   Tuberculosis

The following children are found to have lymphadenopathy. Please select the most likely cause from the list above. Each diagnosis may be used once, more than once or not at all.

1. A 6-month-old baby with severe cradle cap is found to have palpable lymph nodes in the posterior cervical chain. She is otherwise well. At home there is a parrot and they also have some tropical fish.

2. A 6-year-old girl has enlarged and tender lymph nodes in the right axilla and in the right side of the neck. She has been otherwise well, except for a painless lump on her arm that appeared 2 weeks before. At home there is a dog, a cat and a goldfish.

3. A 5-year-old Asian boy has widespread tender lymphadenopathy and a sore throat. Examination also reveals a palpable liver and enlarged tonsils. At home there are several budgerigars.

4. A 3-year-old boy of Ugandan origin presents with weight loss, facial swelling and widespread lymph node enlargement lasting for several weeks. There are no pets at home or infectious contacts, although he often plays near dogs in the playground.

5. A 4-year-old Asian boy has had two recent upper respiratory tract infections and now has a petechial rash. He also has widespread non-tender lymphadenopathy. At home there are tropical fish.

5. THEME: INFECTING ORGANISMS

A   *Escherichia coli*
B   *Haemophilus influenzae* type B (HIB)
C   *Listeria monocytogenes*
D   *Mycoplasma hominis*
E   *Neisseria meningitidis* (meningococcus)
F   *Salmonella enteritidis*
G   *Staphylococcus aureus*
H   *Staphylococcus epidermidis* (coagulase-negative staphylococcus)
I   *Streptococcus pneumoniae* (pneumococcus)
J   *Streptococcus pyogenes* (group A streptococcus)

The children below have presented with an infection. Please select the most likely infecting organism from the above list. Each organism may be used once, more than once or not at all.

1. A 2-year-old with eczema is brought to the GP with worsening of his rash and a high fever. He has a widespead erythematous rash with exudate and golden crusting in some areas.   G

2. A 6-year-old with a Hickman line is undergoing chemotherapy treatment for his neuroblastoma. He presents with a temperature of 38.5 °C, but is systemically well. Peripheral blood cultures are sterile.   H

3. A 5-year-old develops severe abdominal cramps, mild abdominal distension and a temperature of 38.3 °C. He then begins to have severe diarrhoea.   A

4. A 7-year-old girl develops progressive drowsiness with a fever and then has a left-sided focal convulsion. There is no rash.   J

5. A 9-year-old has respiratory distress and a fever. Her chest radiograph shows right lower lobe consolidation.   I

6. THEME: CAUSES OF APNOEA

A   Apnoea of prematurity
B   Behavioural
C   Brain tumour
D   Bronchiolitis
E   Gastro-oesophageal reflux disease
F   Meningitis
G   Non-accidental injury
H   Pertussis
I   Pneumonia
J   Seizure

Each of the children below has presented with apnoea. Please select the most likely cause from the above list. Each option may be used once, more than once or not at all.

1. A 4-week-old boy, born at 28 weeks, is noted to have increasing apnoeas, developing over several hours. Otherwise he seems unchanged, apart from being sleepy and having an unstable temperature.

2. A 5-week-old girl, born at 29 weeks, seems to be doing well. However, over the last week she has been having increasing apnoeas. The change occurred after she was changed from continuous to bolus feeds.

3. A 6-week-old boy, born at 35 weeks, is referred by the GP with poor feeding and apnoeas. He has been previously well, but has been feeding poorly over the last 3 days. There is no fever. On examination, the chest is hyperexpanded.

4. A 7-week-old girl, born at 36 weeks, is seen with a cough, apnoeas and blue spells related to the cough. Her two older brothers both have had 'chesty' coughs for the last 2 weeks.

5. An 8-hour-old baby boy, born at 36 weeks by emergency Caesarian section for fetal distress (and who required resuscitation), is now irritable, with abnormal movements, a high-pitched cry and apnoeas.

7. THEME: USING INVESTIGATIONS

A   CT scan of the brain
B   Full blood count
C   Fundoscopy
D   INR
E   Lumbar puncture
F   MRI scan of the brain
G   Paired urine/blood osmolality
H   Skull radiograph
I   Ultrasound of the brain
J   Urea and electrolytes

Please select the option from the above list that is most appropriate to help make a diagnosis. Each investigation may be used once, more than once or not at all.

1. A 5-year-old has a 2-week history of vomiting in the morning and has now developed a divergent squint.

2. A 5-week-old infant, born at 25 weeks, is found to have a rapidly enlarging head, which is now above the 97th centile.

3. A 4-week-old baby with respiratory syncytial virus (RSV) bronchiolitis has been on intravenous fluids for 3 days, and is now drowsy. His serum Na^+ is 118 mmol/l.

4. Following a road traffic accident, a 3-year-old has become increasingly drowsy. Respiratory and cardiovascular systems are normal. There are no neurological signs.

5. A 6-month-old is admitted after a prolonged focal seizure associated with a temperature. After the seizure she is very drowsy, only able to protect her airway.

8. THEME: CAUSES OF ABDOMINAL DISTENSION

A   Appendicitis
B   Duodenal atresia
C   Hepatomegaly
D   Hirshprung's disease
E   Necrotising enterocolitis
F   Nephrotic syndrome
G   Splenomegaly
H   Peritonitis
I   Pyloric stenosis
J   Wilms' tumour

The children below have presented with abdominal distension. Please select the most likely cause from the above list. Each diagnosis may be used once, more than once or not at all.

1. A 3-year-old has painless abdominal distension that has come on over the last few weeks. There are no other symptoms. Examination is normal except for a ballotable, 10-cm mass to the left of the midline.   *J*

2. A 3-year-old Afro-Caribbean boy is brought urgently by his childminder. He developed abdominal pain and is now hypotensive and unconscious. He has a mass extending from the left costal margin towards the umbilicus.   *G*

3. A 5-year-old has had abdominal pain and fever for the past week. Now her pain is much worse, over the whole abdomen. Examination reveals distension, absent bowel sounds, guarding and rigidity.   *A*

4. A 4-day-old boy has been feeding well, but has progressive abdominal distension. He has not opened his bowels.   *D*

5. A 7-year-old has progressive swelling of his abdomen, as well as around his eyes. He is otherwise well and his abdomen is not tender.   *F*

9. THEME: INVESTIGATION OF RESPIRATORY DISTRESS

A Bronchoscopy
B Chest radiography
C CT chest
D Contrast swallow
E Forced expiratory volume in 1 second (FEV$_1$)
F Noctural oxygen saturation recording
G None of the investigations listed
H Oesophageal pH probe study
I Peak flow
J Sweat test

The children below have presented with respiratory distress. Please select the most useful initial test in their management. Each option may be used once, more than once or not at all.

1. A 2-year-old boy presents with an abrupt onset of coughing and difficulty in breathing. On examination there are reduced breath sounds on the right. B ☐

2. An obese 5-year-old is seen in the Ear, Nose and Throat Clinic with loud snoring at night, sometimes with pauses in his breathing. F ☐

3. A 3-year-old known asthmatic presents with an exacerbation of her asthma. She improves with two puffs of a salbutamol inhaler. E ☐

4. A 6-week-old is seen in the Paediatric Clinic after two episodes of pneumonia requiring antibiotics and admission. Apart from poor weight gain, he is now well. ☐

5. A 9-month-old girl has a 2-day history of coryza and now has inspiratory stridor when agitated. She has no fever and is well oxygenated in air. G ☐

10. THEME: CAUSES OF GROWTH FALTERING

A   Coeliac disease
B   Congenital lactase deficiency
C   Congestive cardiac failure
D   Crohn's disease
E   Cystic fibrosis
F   Gastro-oesophageal reflux
G   Growth hormone deficiency
H   HIV infection
I   Hypothyroidism
J   Neglect

The children below have presented with faltering growth. Please select the most likely cause from the above list. Each diagnosis may be used once, more than once or not at all.

1. A white, 13-month-old boy is now losing weight. His weight gain has fallen off over the last 4 months, although his length is unaffected. He has offensive stools and a distended abdomen. *A*

2. A 6-week-old Afro-Caribbean boy has poor weight gain. He has a liver palpable at 4 cm below the costal margin, a respiratory rate of 45/minute and subcostal recession. He has a poor appetite. *H /c*

3. A 6-year-old Asian girl is becoming short compared with her school friends, although her weight gain is normal for age. Other than this, there are no abnormal physical signs. *G*

4. A white 6-month-old girl has symmetrically poor weight, length and head circumference growth. There are no other abnormal signs, apart from developmental delay. *J*

5. A 3-year-old African boy is admitted with a severe chest infection and persistent diarrhoea. His is noted to have poor weight gain. *B*

11. THEME: FLUID MANAGEMENT OF DIARRHOEA

A   Colloid bolus
B   Dioralyte®
C   Half-strength cow's milk
D   Normal diet
E   0.9% NaCl bolus over 20 minutes
F   0.9% NaCl over 24 hours
G   0.9% NaCl over 48 hours
H   0.45% NaCl/5% dextrose over 24 hours
I   0.45% NaCl/5% dextrose over 48 hours
J   0.45% human albumin solution

The following children have presented to the Emergency Department with diarrhoea. Please select the most appropriate first intervention from the list above. Each option may be used once, more than once or not at all.

1. A 2-year-old has had 2 days of watery stools and vomiting. She has sunken eyes and a dry mouth. Her BP is 92/65 mmHg and her heart rate is 138/bpm. Investigations reveal: Na+ 135 mmol/l, K+ 4.2 mmol/l, urea 7.2 mmol/l.

2. A 4-year-old has had loose stools and vomiting for 4 days. She has sunken eyes and a dry mouth. Her BP is 95/70 mmHg and her heart rate is 135/bpm. Investigations show: Na+ 155 mmol/l, K+ 3.6 mmol/l, urea 9.2 mmol/l.

3. A 3-year-old has had 5 days of loose stools, with at least seven watery motions a day. Her BP is 90/60 mmHg and her heart rate 100/bpm. Investigations show: Na+ 139 mmol/l, K+ 3.9 mmol/l, urea 6.2 mmol/l.

4. A 2-year-old has 2 days of loose stools – three to four each day, with no blood. Her BP is 90/60 mmHg, her heart rate is 105/bpm and she is well perfused.

5. A 4-year-old has 3 days of loose stools – nine or more watery motions a day. His blood pressure is 70/40 mmHg and his heart rate is 155/bpm. Investigations show: Na+ 138 mmol/l, K+ 3.5 mol/l, urea 12 mmol/l.

12. THEME: CAUSES OF ABNORMAL CARDIAC AUSCULTATION FINDINGS

A   Aortic regurgitation
B   Aortic stenosis
C   Atrial septal defect
D   Coarctation of the aorta
E   Mitral regurgitation
F   Mitral stenosis
G   Patent ductus arteriosus
H   Pericardial rub
I   Tricuspid regurgitation
J   Ventricular septal defect

The following children have cardiac murmurs or extra cardiac sounds. Please select the most likely cause from the above list. Each cause may be used once, more than once or not at all.

1. Four days after cardiac surgery for a ventricular septal defect (VSD), a 6-month-old is found to have a scratchy noise in time with his cardiac cycle, but is otherwise doing well.

2. James is seen at a 6-week check. He is thriving and asymtomatic. On examination, he has a grade 2/6 systolic murmur that is loudest below the left clavicle and radiates to the back.

3. A 2-week-old has respiratory distress and tachypnoea. He has a BP of 110/70 mmHg in the right arm and a short systolic murmur just below the left clavicle, grade 2/6, that is radiating to the back.

4. Maggie is seen at a 6-week check. Her weight gain is faltering. She is tachypnoeic, with a liver edge palpable 3 cm below the costal margin. On examination, she is found to have a grade 2/6 pansystolic murmur, loudest at the lower left sternal edge and radiating to the epigastrium.

5. A 7-year-old is seen at the request of the GP, who found a murmur in this otherwise well child. There is fixed splitting of the second heart sound, with a short ejection systolic murmur that is loudest at the left upper sternal edge, with no radiation.

13. THEME: INTERPRETATION OF PAEDIATRIC BLOOD GAS RESULTS

A Asthma
B Barbiturate poisoning
C Bronchiolitis
D Cyanotic congential heart disease
E Diabetic ketoacidosis
F Hypovolaemia due to gastroenteritis
G Inborn error of metabolism
H Paracetamol poisoning
I Pyloric stenosis
J Salicylate poisoning

For the following children and their blood gas results, please select the most likely cause from the above list. Each cause may be used once, more than once or not at all.

1. A 2-day-old child in 100% oxygen with a heart rate of 145/minute, respiratory rate of 27/minute, pH 7.38, $PaCO_2$ 4.5 kPa, PaO_2 4.2 kPa, base excess –2.5 mmol/l, lactate 1.3 mmol/l.

2. A 7-week-old boy in air with vomiting and a heart rate of 180/minute, respiratory rate of 25/minute, pH 7.49, $PaCO_2$ 5.5 kPa, PaO_2 11.3 kPa, base excess +7.5 mmol/l, lactate 2.8 mmol/l.

3. A 6-week-old boy in 30% oxygen with poor feeding, vomiting, a heart rate of 140/minute, respiratory rate of 65/minute, pH 7.19, $PaCO_2$ 10.5 kPa, PaO_2 9.2 kPa, base excess +1.5 mmol/l, lactate 0.9 mmol/l.

4. A 4-day-old baby in air, with poor feeding and floppiness. The heart rate is 145/minute, respiratory rate 40/minute, pH 7.09, $PaCO_2$ 3.3 kPa, PaO_2 9.2 kPa, base excess –16.5 mmol/l, lactate 2.2 mmol/l.

5. A 2-year-old in 35% oxygen with a heart rate of 130/minute, respiratory rate of 35/minute and respiratory distress. Tests reveal: pH 7.43, $PaCO_2$ 3.5 kPa, PaO_2 18.2 kPa, base excess –1.2 mmol/l, lactate 1.1 mmol/l.

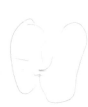

14. THEME: DIAGNOSIS OF LOWER LIMB DISORDERS

A   Congenital dislocation of the hip
B   Diplegic cerebral palsy
C   Duchenne's muscular dystrophy
D   Fracture of the neck of femur
E   Osteomyelitis of the femur
F   Osteosarcoma of the femur
G   Perthes' disease (avascular necrosis of the hip)
H   Sciatica
I   Septic arthritis
J   Slipped femoral epiphysis

For the following children please select the most likely diagnosis from the above list. Each diagnosis may be used once, more than once or not at all.

1. A 6-month-old girl is not moving her left leg, holding it rigidly in flexion and external rotation. She has a fever and a raised neutrophil count.

2. A normal, very active 12-year-old boy has been limping increasingly for the last 2 weeks and has pain in the right thigh. He cannot remember if anything precipitated the problem. His true leg length is equal, but the apparent length of the right leg is reduced.

3. A 3-year-old girl has an asymmetrical gait. A full neurological examination is normal. She has limited abduction of the left hip, with a shortened apparent leg length on the same side.

4. A 3-month-old baby has a fever and is not moving her right leg. Examination of the leg reveals a swollen and tender thigh, with reduced movement of the right hip.

5. A child aged 21 months has been referred with delay in walking – he was not walking at 19 months, although he has now started to take a few steps. On examination, he has a symmetrical but unsteady gait. Neurological examination is normal, but he has apparent hypertrophy of his calves.

15. THEME: CAUSES OF ABNORMAL BREATH SOUNDS

A Asthma
B Bronchiolitis
C Inhaled foreign body in left main bronchus
D Inhaled foreign body in right main bronchus
E Laryngotracheobronchitis (croup)
F Left pneumothorax
G Left-sided pneumonia
H Pulmonary oedema
I Right pneumothorax
J Right-sided pneumonia

The following children have been examined. For each, select the most likely diagnosis from the list above. Each diagnosis may be used once, more than once or not at all.

1. A white, 12-week-old boy has a respiratory rate of 60 breaths/minute, subcostal recession and tracheal tug, and a prolonged expiratory phase. Auscultation reveals bilateral expiratory crackles and wheeze.

2. A 6-year-old asthmatic child has a respiratory rate of 40 breaths/minute and subcostal and intercostal recession. He is hyperexpanded on the right and his trachea is deviated to the left. Auscultation reveals normal breath sounds on the left with reduced sounds on the right.

3. An 8-year-old child with nephrotic syndrome has a respiratory rate of 32 breaths/minute, subcostal recession and tracheal tug. Auscultation reveals bilateral late-inspiratory fine crepitations, especially in the lung bases.

4. A 2-year-old has deteriorated after an upper respiratory tract infection. Now she has a respiratory rate of 45 breaths/minute, with subcostal recession and tracheal tug. Her trachea is central. Expansion is reduced on the left. Auscultation reveals left-sided inspiratory crackles.

5. A 2-year-old boy with difficulty breathing has a respiratory rate of 40 breaths/minute, subcostal recession and tracheal tug. His trachea is deviated to the left and he has reduced expansion on the left. Auscultation reveals absent breath sounds on the left and normal sounds on the right.

CHAPTER 6

Radiology

1. THEME: MUSCULOSKELETAL RADIOGRAPHS I – RADIOLOGICAL DIAGNOSIS
2. THEME: MUSCULOSKELETAL RADIOGRAPHS II – CLINICAL DIAGNOSIS
3. THEME: MUSCULOSKELETAL RADIOGRAPHS III – CLINICAL SCENARIOS

1–3 A

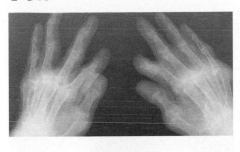

1–3 B

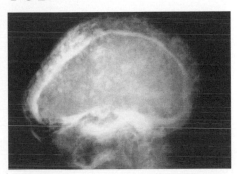

1–3 C

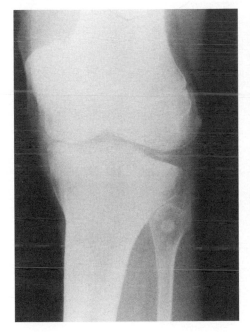

1–3 D

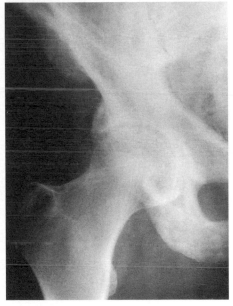

THEMES 1–3: pages 141, 142

1. THEME: MUSCULOSKELETAL RADIOGRAPHS I –
   RADIOLOGICAL DIAGNOSIS
2. THEME: MUSCULOSKELETAL RADIOGRAPHS II –
   CLINICAL DIAGNOSIS
3. THEME: MUSCULOSKELETAL RADIOGRAPHS III –
   CLINICAL SCENARIOS

1–3 E

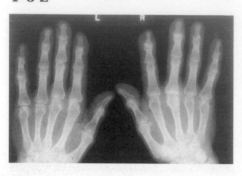

1–3 F

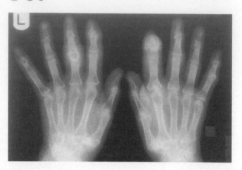

1–3 G

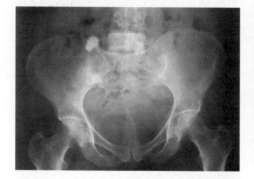

1–3 H

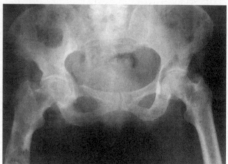

THEMES 1–3: pages 141, 142

1. THEME: MUSCULOSKELETAL RADIOGRAPHS I – RADIOLOGICAL DIAGNOSIS
2. THEME: MUSCULOSKELETAL RADIOGRAPHS II – CLINICAL DIAGNOSIS
3. THEME: MUSCULOSKELETAL RADIOGRAPHS III – CLINICAL SCENARIOS

1–3 I

1–3 J

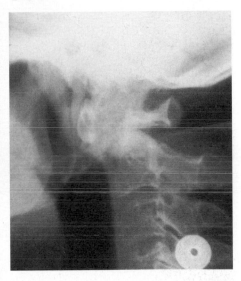

THEMES 1–3: pages 141, 142

4. THEME: GASTROENTEROLOGICAL RADIOLOGY I – CLINICAL DIAGNOSIS
5. THEME: GASTROENTEROLOGICAL RADIOLOGY II – CLINICAL SCENARIOS
6. THEME: GASTROENTEROLOGICAL RADIOLOGY III – RADIOLOGICAL DIAGNOSIS

4–6 A

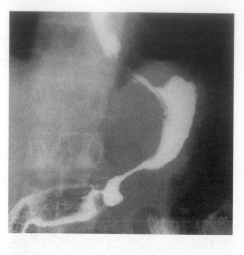

4–6 B

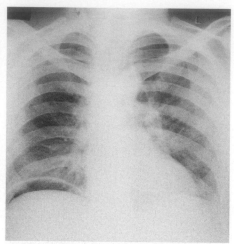

4–6 C

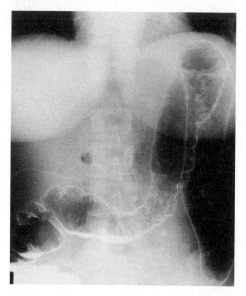

4–6 D

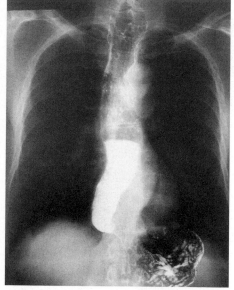

THEMES 4–6: pages 143, 144, 145

4. THEME: GASTROENTEROLOGICAL RADIOLOGY I – CLINICAL DIAGNOSIS
5. THEME: GASTROENTEROLOGICAL RADIOLOGY II – CLINICAL SCENARIOS
6. THEME: GASTROENTEROLOGICAL RADIOLOGY III – RADIOLOGICAL DIAGNOSIS

4–6 E

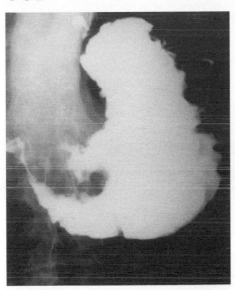

4–6 F

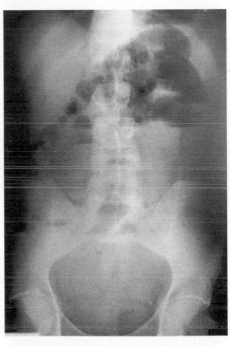

4–6 G

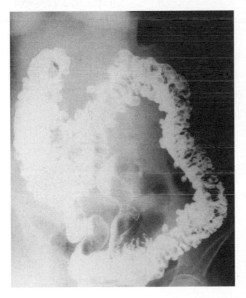

4–6 H

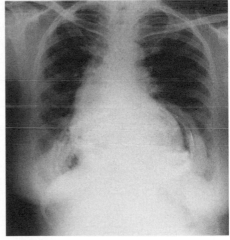

THEMES 4–6: pages 143, 144, 145

4. THEME: GASTROENTEROLOGICAL RADIOLOGY I –
CLINICAL DIAGNOSIS
5. THEME: GASTROENTEROLOGICAL RADIOLOGY II –
CLINICAL SCENARIOS
6. THEME: GASTROENTEROLOGICAL RADIOLOGY III –
RADIOLOGICAL DIAGNOSIS

4–6 I

4–6 J

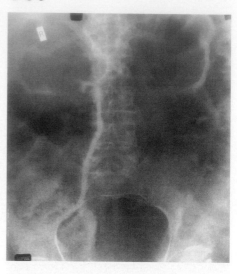

THEMES 4–6: pages 143, 144, 145

1. THEME: MUSCULOSKELETAL RADIOGRAPHS I – RADIOLOGICAL DIAGNOSIS

*Using the radiographic images **A–J on pages 135–137**, please match the radiological diagnoses below with the correct image. You may use the images once, more than once or not at all. There may be more than one correct image for each of the diagnoses.*

1. Lytic bone lesions. B, H ☐

2. Intra-articular calcification. D, A ☐

3. Cortical thickening. B ☐

4. 'Bamboo spine'. J ☐

5. Subluxation. F ☐

6. Sclerotic bone lesion. A ☐

2. THEME: MUSCULOSKELETAL RADIOGRAPHS II – CLINICAL DIAGNOSIS

*Using the radiographic images **A–J on pages 135–137**, please match the diagnoses shown below with the correct image. You may use the images once, more than once or not at all. There may be more than one image appropriate for each of the diagnoses.*

1. Ankylosing spondylitis. ☐

2. Tophaceous gout. ☐

3. Metastatic secondary deposits. ☐

4. Paget's disease of bone. ☐

5. Osteoarthritis. ☐

6. Pyrophosphate arthropathy. ☐

3. THEME: MUSCULOSKELETAL RADIOGRAPHS III – CLINICAL SCENARIOS

*The patients below have all presented with skeletal or rheumatological conditions. Using the radiographic images **A–J on pages 135–137**, please match the presentations with the correct image. You may use each image once, more than once or not at all.*

1. A 42-year-old woman with long-standing rheumatoid arthritis is admitted for a total knee replacement. She tells the FY2 doctor that she has had 'pins and needles' and numbness in all four of her limbs and is finding it increasingly difficult to move about. A routine radiograph ordered by the anaesthetist in the pre-admissions clinic confirms the diagnosis.

2. A 79-year-old man is seen by his GP with a severe, acutely painful and swollen monoarthritis. He improves with non-steroidal anti-inflammatory drugs (NSAIDs). The diagnosis is subsequently confirmed by a radiograph of the affected joint and intra-articular aspiration, which demonstrates weakly positive birefringent crystals under polarised light.

3. An 86-year-old man is seen by his GP with reduced mobility secondary to hip and pelvic pain. Routine investigations confirm normal serum calcium, phosphate and γGT, with a grossly elevated alkaline phosphatase.

4. A 67-year-old man presents to his GP with a 2-month history of worsening back pain and episodic haematuria. The diagnosis is subsequently confirmed by a prostate-specific antigen (PSA) level of 1460 IU/l, radiographs and a positive bone scan.

5. A 41-year-old man with long-standing arthritis, which in the past has responded to physiotherapy and simple analgesia, presents to his GP with increasing stiffness of his lower back and exertional dyspnoea. Of note in his family history, his maternal grandmother had inflammatory bowel disease and his mother had psoriasis.

4. THEME: GASTROENTEROLOGICAL RADIOLOGY I – CLINICAL DIAGNOSIS

*The patients below have all presented with gastroenterological conditions. Using the radiographic images **A–J on pages 138–140**, please match the diagnoses with the correct image. You may use the images once, more than once or not at all. There may be more than one image appropriate for each of the diagnoses.*

1. Achalasia.

2. A hiatus hernia.

3. A malignant lesion.

4. Small-bowel obstruction.

5. Inflammatory bowel disease.

6. Diverticulosis.

5. THEME: GASTROENTEROLOGICAL RADIOLOGY II – CLINICAL SCENARIOS

*The patients below have all presented with gastroenterological conditions. Using the radiographic images **A–J on pages 138–140**, please match the presentations with the correct image. You may use each image once, more than once or not at all.*

1. A 24-year-old woman presents 24 hours after a routine, day-case, laparoscopic procedure complaining of bloating and nausea. On examination, she looks well and is apyrexial and her routine observations are normal. Her abdomen is slightly distended and mildly tender, but there are good bowel sounds with no evidence of peritonism. Radiological investigation reveals an expected abnormality.

2. A 63-year-old man presents to his GP with a 4-month history of weight loss and intermittent but worsening constipation. His initial investigations show: haemoglobin 7.9 g/dl, MCV 65 fl, WCC 9.4 × 10⁹/l, platelets 443 × 10⁹/l; total bilirubin 32.6 μmol/l, albumin 31 g/l, ALT 132 IU/l, AST 102 IU/l, alkaline phosphatase 788 IU/l.

3. An 81-year-old woman presents to her GP with a 4-month history of intermittent constipation, weight loss and occasional bright-red blood per rectum. She refuses colonoscopy but a benign diagnosis is confirmed radiologically and she improves with the addition of Milpar® and senna and by increasing the fibre in her diet.

4. A 63-year-old man presents to the Emergency Department with a 36-hour history of severe, generalised abdominal pain and profuse vomiting. Of note in his past surgical history he has had an appendicectomy and an aortic aneurysm repair. On examination, he is clammy, with a blood pressure of 100/50 mmHg, pulse 120 bpm and regular, capillary blood glucose of 12.6 mmol/l and oxygen saturation 94% on air. Abdominal examination reveals a distended abdomen with no organomegaly. Bowel sounds are 'very active and distant'.

5. A 37-year-old woman presents to her GP with increasingly severe lower thoracic dysphagia. She has found it necessary to eat only small amounts at a time and these need to be washed down with increasing amounts of fluid. More recently, she has regurgitated several undigested meals.

6. THEME: GASTROENTEROLOGICAL RADIOLOGY III – RADIOLOGICAL DIAGNOSIS

The patients below have all presented with gastroenterological conditions. Using the radiographic images A–J on pages 130–140, please match the radiological diagnosis with the correct image. You may use the images once, more than once or not at all. There may be more than one image appropriate for each of the diagnoses.

1. An 'apple core' lesion.

2. 'Lead piping' of the large bowel.

3. Linitis plastica.

4. A 'bird's beak' lesion.

5. Pathologically dilated bowel loops.

6. Pneumoperitoneum.

CHAPTER **7**

Surgery

1. THEME: INVESTIGATION OF ABDOMINAL PAIN

A   Chest and abdominal radiographs
B   Colonoscopy
C   CT scan
D   Diagnostic laparoscopy
E   Gastroscopy
F   General abdominal ultrasound
G   Laparotomy
H   None – regular clinical review
I   Pelvic (transvaginal) ultrasound scan
J   Proctosigmoidoscopy

The following scenarios describe patients with various causes of abdominal pain. Assuming that they have undergone resuscitation and basic investigation, please choose from the list above the most appropriate next step in management. Each option may be used once, more than once or not at all.

1. A 56-year-old woman presents with intermittent post-prandial right upper quadrant pain with some associated dyspepsia.

2. A 69-year-old hypertensive smoker presents with a 3-hour history of sudden onset of worsening lower back pain and bilateral lower limb paralysis.

3. A 24-year-old man presents with sudden-onset and rapidly increasing epigastric pain. On examination, he is dehydrated, tachycardic and has widespread abdominal peritonism.

4. An 80-year-old woman presents with a 24-hour history of absolute constipation and lower abdominal pain. On examination, her abdomen is grossly distended.

5. An 18-year-old woman presents with a 14-hour history of right iliac fossa pain, associated with nausea and vomiting. On examination, there is tenderness and guarding in the right iliac fossa. She reports, however, that her pain is similar to what she experienced 1 year ago when she had a torted ovarian cyst and required surgery.

2. THEME: FAECAL INCONTINENCE

A   Acute gastroenteritis
B   Colorectal carcinoma
C   Extrarectal or rectovaginal fistula
D   Faecal impaction
E   Inflammatory bowel disease
F   Pudendal neuropathy
G   Sphincter disruption
H   Spinal cord lesion
I   Systemic neuropathology

The following patients have all presented with faecal incontinence. From the above list please choose the most appropriate cause. Each option may be used once, more than once or not at all

1. A 26-year-old woman is referred by her GP with passive faecal incontinence, which has she has had since the birth of her child 3 months ago.

2. A 68-year-old man presents with new onset of faecal incontinence. He has been previously fit and well, but now describes passing loose stools with increased frequency and with some mucus.

3. A 60-year-old woman with four children presents with a 3-year history of worsening urge faecal incontinence. She had two prolonged, instrumented deliveries.

4. A 92-year-old woman who lives in a nursing home has constant problems with faecal soiling and has to wear incontinence pads day and night.

5. A 45-year-old man presents with a 24-hour history of severe, cramping lower abdominal pain associated with nausea and diarrhoea (severe urgency, ten stools a day, very watery). He has an episode of incontinence while waiting in the GP surgery.

3. THEME: GROIN LUMPS

A Ectopic testis
B False aneurysm
C Femoral artery aneurysm
D Femoral hernia
E Hydrocele of the spermatic cord
F Inguinal hernia
G Inguinal lymphadenopathy
H Psoas abscess
I Psoas bursa
J Saphena varix

The following patients all present with a lump in the groin. For each scenario please select the most appropriate diagnosis from the above list. Each diagnosis may be used once, more than once or not at all.

1. A 24-year-old man notices a lump in his groin after lifting a heavy load. On examination, you find a reducible lump that lies above and medial to the pubic tubercle.

2. A 28-year-old man has noticed small painful lumps in both groins that have been present for some weeks. On questioning, he gives a history of some dysuria and penile discharge.

3. A 36-year-old Asian immigrant presents to the Emergency Department with a tender, fluctuant mass in his left femoral triangle. He gives a history of night sweats, weight loss and a painful left hip. On examination, there is pain on passive extension of the hip.

4. A 78-year-old woman attends the Emergency Department with drowsiness and confusion. Her husband reports a 12-hour history of vomiting and abdominal pain. On examination, she is clearly dehydrated, her abdomen is distended and she has obstructed bowel sounds. More detailed assessment reveals a small painful swelling in her right groin crease.

5. A 62-year-old patient with claudication returns to the ward from the Vascular Assessment Laboratory after having an angiogram of his lower limbs. The nurse is concerned about a swelling in his left groin. On closer examination you note a firm mass with a transmissible pulse.

4. THEME: POSTOPERATIVE HYPOXIA

A   Adult respiratory distress syndrome
B   Basal atelectasis
C   Bronchospasm
D   Lobar collapse
E   Opiate overdose
F   Pleural effusion
G   Pneumonia
H   Pneumothorax
I   Pulmonary embolism
J   Pulmonary oedema
K   Upper airway obstruction

The following are descriptions of patients with postoperative hypoxia. Please select the most appropriate diagnosis from the above list. The options may be used once, more than once or not at all.

1. A 35-year-old woman undergoes a total thyroidectomy. Two hours post-operatively she develops severe respiratory distress.

2. A 62-year-old woman undergoes a sigmoid colectomy for left-sided colonic carcinoma. She is given an epidural for pain relief, but this becomes dislodged. On day 1 after surgery she is dyspnoeic, with a rapid pulse and mild pyrexia. Auscultation reveals reduced breath sounds at the left base. The arterial blood gases are: pH 7.35, PaO_2 9.6 kPa, $PaCO_2$ 5.0 kPa. She has a non-productive cough.

3. A 74-year-old man with a previous history of ischaemic heart disease undergoes an anterior resection for rectal carcinoma. On day 4 after the operation he becomes severely dyspnoeic and tachypnoeic, but is apyrexial. Auscultation reveals bilateral fine crepitations. The arterial blood gases are: pH 7.35, PaO_2 8.0 kPa, $PaCO_2$ 5.5 kPa.

4. A 59-year-old man undergoes a palliative bypass of an unresectable gastric carcinoma. Several days later he is dyspnoeic and mildly tachycardic, but is apyrexial. Auscultation reveals absent breath sounds at the left base and reduced left-sided vocal resonance. The arterial blood gases are: pH 7.37, PaO_2 10.1 kPa, $PaCO_2$ 6.0 kPa. His serum albumin is 20 g/l.

5. A 43-year-old woman is being treated for severe acute pancreatitis. Over the past 48 hours she has become increasingly dyspnoeic and tachycardic. Auscultation reveals bilateral fine crepitations. The arterial blood gases are: pH 7.37, PaO_2 8.2 kPa, $PaCO_2$ 4.9 kPa. Chest radiographs shows bilateral diffuse infiltrates.

5. THEME: POSTOPERATIVE OLIGURIA

A   Acute renal failure
B   Cardiogenic shock
C   Dehydration
D   Haemorrhagic shock
E   Increased ADH secretion
F   Obstructed urinary catheter
G   Sepsis
H   Ureteric injury
I   Urinary retention

The above are all causes of postoperative oliguria. For the following scenarios please pick the most appropriate answer from the list. Each option may be used once, more than once or not at all.

1. A 64-year-old man has undergone elective surgery for repair of his aortic aneurysm. He is recovering on the High Dependency Unit when the nurses call you to inform you that he has only passed 5–10 ml/hour of urine for the past 4 hours, despite catheter flushing. On examination, you find that his abdomen is distended, his BP is 90/55 mmHg and his pulse is 105 bpm.

2. A 60-year-old diabetic man is recovering from a left femoro-popliteal bypass. The nurses call you to let you know that he has failed to pass more than 5 ml/hour of urine for the past 3 hours. They have been giving him Gaviscon® for 'indigestion', which has not settled. On examination you find that he is a pale and sweaty, his BP is 95/60 mmHg and his pulse is 98 pm. The bandages covering his operative wound are minimally bloodstained and his thigh, although slightly swollen, is soft. Two fluid challenges (Gelofusin®, 250 ml each) fail to improve his BP.

3. A 66-year-old man undergoes a left hemicolectomy for cancer. Twelve hours post-operatively, you are called because his urine output has been <50 ml/hour for the last 4 hours. The vital signs are otherwise stable and normal and the patient is comfortable. He responds to fluid challenges.

4. A 56-year-old man undergoes a left hemicolectomy for cancer. Twelve hours post-operatively, you are called because his urine output has been 25 ml, 20 ml and 10 ml over the last 3 hours and he is now anuric. Vital signs are otherwise stable and normal.

6. THEME: ADVANCES RELATED TO SURGERY

A   Christian Theodor Billroth
B   Astley Cooper
C   Alexander Fleming
D   William Halstead
E   John Hunter
F   Emil Kocher
G   Karl Landsteiner
H   Joseph Lister
I   James Paget
J   John Snow
K   Frederick Treves

The following are descriptions of significant discoveries that are linked to the modern practice of surgery. Please select the name linked with each discovery from the above list. Each name may be used once, more than once, or not at all.

1.   His name is eponymously associated a breast and bone disorder. ☐

2.   He made contributions to development of anaesthesia (as well in the field of the epidemiology of cholera). ☐

3.   He made contributions to development of blood transfusion. ☐

4.   A German-born professor of surgery in Vienna. Best known for his contributions to gastric surgery. The first surgeon to suggest a formal structure to surgical training. ☐

5.   An American surgeon who was the first to use rubber gloves. He invented operations for inguinal hernia and mastectomy. ☐

7. THEME: ENTERAL AND PARENTERAL NUTRITION

A   Eating and drinking
B   Elemental diet
C   Feeding jejunostomy
D   Fortisips®/Ensure®
E   Intravenous nutrition
F   Low-volume, low-electrolyte diet
G   Modular diet
H   Nasogastric feeding
I   Nasojejunal feeding
J   Peptide diet
K   Percutaneous endoscopic gastrostomy (PEG) feeding

The above are all examples of types and routes of nutritional support. For the following statements please choose the most appropriate option from the list. Each option may be used once, more than once or not at all.

1. The best route for early postoperative feeding after oesophagectomy.

2. A patient with chronic renal failure who is managed by continuous ambulatory peritoneal dialysis.

3. The best route for nutrition in a patient who has had a stroke and who will require feeding for the foreseeable future (ie more than 4 weeks).

4. A patient who has had a superior mesenteric arterial infarction is recovering postoperatively. The surgical notes state that only 95 cm of bowel was viable at operation and a small-bowel stoma has been formed. The patient requires nutritional support.

5. A patient with predicted acute severe pancreatitis is transferred to the High Dependency Unit. You are asked by 'enlightened' staff to make a plan for ongoing nutritional support.

8. THEME: TYPES OF SHOCK

A   Anaphylactic
B   Cardiogenic
C   Haemorrhagic
D   Endocrine-related
E   Neurogenic
F   Non-haemorrhagic hypovolaemic
G   Septic
H   Spinal

The following are descriptions of shock. Please select the most appropriate diagnosis from the above list. Each diagnosis may be used once, more than once or not at all.

1. A 28-year-old man falls from a ladder and sustains a displaced spinal fracture with cord transaction at T12/L1. Other injuries include bilateral wrist fractures and a minor head injury. His BP remains low despite fluid resuscitation and his pulse is 60 bpm.

2. A 32-year-old man is stabbed in the left side of the chest. Initial assessment reveals engorged neck veins, a respiratory rate of 30/minute, a pulse of 120 bpm and a BP of 80/40 mmHg, despite attempts at fluid resuscitation. On auscultation, the heart sounds are muffled.

3. A 72-year-old man presents with sudden onset of severe central abdominal pain. On examination, he is very anxious, with a respiratory rate of 33 breaths/minute, pulse 120 bpm and BP 90/40 mmHg. He has passed 15 ml of urine since he was catheterised 1 hour ago. Both femoral pulses are only faintly palpable.

4. A 61-year-old man becomes acutely confused on day 3 after an abdominal aortic aneurysm repair. Examination reveals: temperature 38 °C, respiratory rate 36 breaths/minute, pulse 110 bpm and BP 90/40 mmHg, despite attempts at fluid resuscitation. He has passed a negligible volume of urine since he was catheterised 1 hour ago. Ironically, his peripheries are warm to the touch.

5. A 26-year-old man is knocked off his bike by a lorry. He is intubated at the scene because he has a head injury, and a chest drain has been inserted for a right-sided pneumothorax (this has drained 50 ml blood). A pelvic radiograph shows pubic rami fractures and he has an open fracture of the right femur. While awaiting further investigation, he is given cefuroxime and metronidazole as part of the management for his open fracture. Shortly afterwards, his observations are: pulse 150 bpm, BP 80/40 mmHg.

9. THEME: MANAGEMENT DECISIONS IN TRAUMA CARE

A   Abdominal radiograph
B   Angiography
C   Chest drain
D   Chest, pelvic and lateral cervical spine radiographs
E   CT scan
F   Diagnostic peritoneal lavage (DPL)
G   Emergency laparotomy
H   Emergency thoracotomy
I   Focused assessment with sonography for trauma (FAST) scan
J   Local wound exploration
K   Resuscitation (Emergency-Room) thoracotomy
L   Transfer to specialist unit

In the following scenario, a patient has arrived in the Emergency Department after a serious road traffic accident. Sequential management decisions will be required. From the list above, choose the most appropriate answer. Each option may be used once, more than once or not at all.

A 28-year-old cyclist has been brought into the Emergency Department after being knocked off his bicycle by a lorry. He has bruising to his left flank and is complaining of abdominal pain. A primary survey (A to E) is performed and resuscitation started. He is conscious and maintaining a BP of 110/75 mmHg, a pulse of 120 bpm and a respiratory rate of 30 breaths/minute.

1. What is your first investigation? This investigation demonstrates no abnormality. He responds to fluid resuscitation (BP 120/80 mmHg, pulse 96 bpm). □

2. What test would you perform next? This test demonstrates some free fluid in the abdomen. □

3. He remains haemodynamically stable without further fluid resuscitation. What would you plan to do next? □

4. While contemplating the test you were planning in question 3, however, he becomes very unstable again (systolic BP 85 mmHg, pulse 135 bpm).What would you do now? □

10. THEME: INVESTIGATION AND MANAGEMENT OF GASTROINTESTINAL DISEASE

A   Angiography
B   Barium meal/barium follow-through
C   Bidirectional endoscopy
D   Capsule endoscopy
E   Colonoscopy
F   CT scan
G   Double-contrast barium enema
H   Emergency surgery
I   Flexible sigmoidoscopy
J   Oesophagogastroduodenoscopy (OGD) and adrenaline (epinephrine) injection
K   OGD and banding
L   OGD and sclerotherapy
M   Proctosigmoidoscopy
N   Red-cell radionucleotide scanning

The above are all methods of investigating or treating gastrointestinal bleeding. For the following scenarios please pick the most appropriate answer from the list. Each option may be used once, more than once or not at all. (In these scenarios, it is taken for granted that all the patients have already been appropriately resuscitated.)

1. A 66-year-old woman presents with a 3-year history of constipation and vague lower abdominal discomfort. There is no rectal bleeding. Rectal and abdominal examination are unremarkable; sigmoidoscopy is limited by hard faeces.

2. A 57-year-old man presents with significant haematemesis and melaena. After resuscitation he undergoes upper gastrointestinal endoscopy. This shows an actively bleeding duodenal ulcer with a visible vessel at its base.

3. A 30-year-old man presents to the Emergency Department with a short history of bright-red bleeding per rectum. On questioning, he has a long history of noticing blood on the toilet paper and occasionally in the toilet pan. He is otherwise well. His haemoglobin is 13.7 g/dl.

4. A 47-year-old man presents to his GP with lethargy. He has no gastrointestinal symptoms. Investigations show: no abnormalities on urine dipstick, haemoglobin 8.2 g/dl, MCV 65.4 fl, U&Es normal.

5. A 67-year-old woman presents with a history of melaena that is increasing in frequency. Her last few motions have also contained fresh, dark-red blood. Her haemoglobin is 10.9 g/dl. An upper gastrointestinal endoscopy is normal and an unprepared colonoscopy does not clearly identify a source of acute bleeding. Despite adequate fluid resuscitation, she continues to be haemodynamically unstable, with a repeat haemoglobin of 7.0 g/dl. A blood transfusion has been commenced.

ANSWERS

ANSWERS TO CHAPTER – GASTROENTEROLOGY

1. ANATOMY OF THE ALIMENTARY TRACT

1. **H – Second part of the duodenum**
   These Brunner's glands of the duodenum are characteristic. The C-shaped formation of the duodenum surrounds the head, body and uncinate process of the pancreas, and is centred at the level of the second lumbar vertebra.

2. **G – Pylorus**
   This is the transpyloric plane. The stomach has circular, longitudinal and oblique muscle layers, the circular layer producing the prominent pyloric sphincter.

3. **I – Sigmoid colon mesentery**
   The V-shaped root of the sigmoid mesentery also crosses the left common iliac artery and the left sacroiliac joint. The small-intestinal mesentery passes from the duodenojejunal flexure at the level of the second lumbar vertebra, obliquely downwards to the right sacroiliac joint, crossing the left psoas muscle, the aorta, inferior vena cava, the right gonadal vessels, the right psoas and the right ureter.

4. **B – Ascending colon**
   The ascending colon overlies the iliacus and quadratus lumborum, and is overlaid anteriorly by the peritoneum and small intestine. The descending colon in addition lies on the diaphragm above and curves medially onto the psoas muscle inferiorly.

5. **F – Jejunum**
   The jejunum has prominent villi for absorption, in contrast to the duodenum and colon where they are absent.

2. VOMITING

1. **C – Drug therapy**
   Vomiting in this case is due to digoxin toxicity. Hypokalaemia secondary to the use of diuretic predisposes to digoxin toxicity. Vomiting itself is another cause of hypokalaemia, which can aggravate the situation. Patients are usually nauseated and have a slow heart rate.

2. **F – Gastroenteritis due to *Staphylococcus aureus***
   The short history in this case is typical of staphylococcal gastroenteritis caused by preformed enterotoxin (an exotoxin) from food contaminated with *Staphylococcus aureus*. The vomiting starts shortly after ingestion of the offending dish (a wide variety of foodstuffs can be contaminated). Other causative organisms of vomiting-predominant food poisoning include *Bacillus cereus*, but the history is typically shorter (1–2 hours) and symptoms start much later after ingestion of the contaminated food (approximately 8 hours after ingestion). Vomiting also occurs with enteric infections with bacteria such

as *Salmonella*, *Campylobacter* and *Shigella*, but the predominant symptoms in such cases are invariably lower abdominal pain, diarrhoea or dysentery.

3.   **G – Gastric outflow obstruction**
Gastric outflow obstruction has been caused in this case by neonatal pyloric stenosis. This patient is the right age for this (3–6 weeks), and has the characteristic history of this disorder (projectile vomiting after each meal). The finding of the so-called 'pyloric tumour' caused by pyloric contraction during feeding provides further confirmation. The disorder is due to hypertrophy of circular muscle of the pyloric region of the stomach. The baby is classically well and seeking more feed after vomiting but dehydration and severe electrolyte disturbances (especially acid-base disorder and hypokalaemia) will eventually arise. The condition is treated surgically with a Ramstedt pyloromyotomy.

4.   **I – Small-intestinal obstruction**
This is the classic clinical description of a patient presenting with small-bowel obstruction – colicky, central abdominal pain, distension, nausea and vomiting (eventually bile-stained). In this woman's case, the cause is probably adhesions secondary to her previous intra-abdominal inflammation/sepsis. In contrast, gastric outflow obstruction does not cause bilious vomiting and large-intestinal obstruction is characterised by lower abdominal colic and constipation, with vomiting (faeculant) being a later feature.

5.   **A – Acute abdomen**
This is a case of acute abdomen, probably appendicitis. Acute inflammation affecting any part of the gastrointestinal tract will lead to a localised ileus (or generalised ileus in the case of generalised peritonitis) and to nausea and vomiting. Common examples include pancreatitis, cholecystitis and appendicitis.

NB: A complete overview of all the causes of vomiting (not possible in one EMQ) should include the following:

● Central – intracranial, labyrinthine
● Metabolic and endocrine – uraemia, pregnancy, diabetes
● Iatrogenic – cancer chemotherapy, digoxin, opiates
● Obstructive – any level (see above)
● Mucosal – appendicitis, gastritis, cholecystitis.

3.   HAEMATEMESIS

1.   **B – Gastric erosions**
The most likely cause is gastric erosions. Stress ulceration leading to erosions of the stomach (and to some extent also of the duodenum) is a complication of significant burns (Curling's ulcer), as well as other traumatic injuries, systemic sepsis, intracranial lesions (Cushing's ulcer) and organ failure (eg uraemia). The risk of bleeding can be reduced by giving a mucosa-protecting agent such as sucralfate or prophylactic antacid treatments (eg ranitidine). These agents are therefore commonly used in an intensive-care environment.

2. **J – Zollinger–Ellison syndrome**
    Zollinger–Ellison syndrome is a rare disorder caused by a gastrin-secreting tumour found either in the islet cells of the pancreas or in the duodenal wall. The release of gastrin stimulates the production of large quantities of hydrochloric acid in the gastric antrum, leading to predominantly distal (duodenal) ulceration. Diagnosis is suspected in patients with recurrent peptic ulceration and facilitated by the measurement of persistently high serum gastrin levels and tumour imaging by ultrasonography, computed tomography (CT) or angiography. Acid secretion can be suppressed to some extent by proton-pump inhibitors (eg lansoprazole).

3. **G – Oesophageal varices**
    Although a full history is not available, the history of massive haematemesis in combination with the blood investigation results, with a raised mean corpuscular volume (MCV, due to alcohol-induced bone marrow toxicity) and a raised international normalised ratio (INR, due to severe hepatic dysfunction) makes oesophageal varices the likely diagnosis. Varices are caused by portal hypertension, usually secondary to cirrhosis of the liver. Following initial resuscitation an emergency upper gastrointestinal endoscopy will confirm the presence of varices and might also (in skilled hands) allow therapeutic intervention (banding or injection sclerotherapy). Attempts should also be made to correct the coagulopathy urgently (vitamin K injections, fresh-frozen plasma). The mortality from variceal bleeding is very high. In life-threatening situations, a Sengstaken–Blakemore tube can be used for balloon tamponade of the bleeding.

4. **A – Gastric carcinoma**
    A man of this age is likely to have a gastric carcinoma, as evidenced by the history of symptoms such as dyspepsia, nausea, anorexia, weight loss and, in particular, early satiety (a feeling of fullness after eating small amounts of food). Chronic blood loss over some time is suggested by the finding of a microcytic anaemia.

5. **H – Mallory-Weiss tear**
    The correct answer is Mallory-Weiss tear, as evidenced by the classic history. Bleeding is from mucosal vessels damaged by a tear in the mucosa at the gastro-oesophageal junction that occurs as a result of repeated retching/vomiting (almost always in practice due to alcohol excess). The bleeding is usually only slight to moderate and is nearly always self limiting (hence the normal blood results).

4. CONSTIPATION

1. **A – Carcinoma of the colon/rectum**
    This diagnosis must always be considered in someone presenting with a short history of change in bowel habit to constipation. The diagnosis is further suggested by the passage of mucus and tenesmus (especially with low rectal tumours), which is the disabling feeling of needing to pass stool but being unable to do so.

2. **H – Iatrogenic (drug therapy)**
    This patient's constipation has been caused by prescribed medical therapy. A number of antipsychotic treatments (eg chlorpromazine) have anticholinergic side-effects, mediated by their antagonism of the muscarinic effects of acetylcholine and therefore including effects on the gastrointestinal tract (decreased motility and gland

secretions – hence the dry mouth), the bladder (inability to pass urine), eyes (blurring of vision) and many others. While some psychiatric disorders are clearly associated with constipation (eg depression) a causal relationship is less clear.

3. **J – Simple constipation**
Constipation is the second most common gastrointestinal symptom in the developed world after dyspepsia. In the majority, the symptom is mild and self-limiting. Low fluid intake, a low-fibre diet, and lack of exercise and mobility are all factors that contribute to simple constipation. In addition, it is a common accompaniment of ageing. Elderly inpatients such as the woman described here are very commonly affected by constipation for these reasons. Treatment should aim at reversing the above causative factors where possible but laxatives are usually required, at least in the short term.

4. **B – Chronic idiopathic constipation**
The long history from an early age and the female sex make an organic diagnosis very unlikely. When no organic cause can be found, the problem is described as 'idiopathic'. The majority of such patients have intractable symptoms which do not respond to simple laxative therapy. The group can be further divided by physiological studies into those with a delay in transit in all or part of the colon (slow-transit constipation), those with abnormalities of rectal evacuation and those with no abnormality ('constipation-predominant irritable bowel syndrome'). The cause or causes of such disorders are unclear.

5. **F – Hypercalcaemia**
The diagnosis can be deduced indirectly. This man is likely, on the basis of the history, to have a carcinoma of the bronchus (cough and haemoptysis). Hypercalcaemia can occur quite commonly with lung cancer due to malignant infiltration of bone (osteolysis and calcium release) or due to ectopic secretion by the tumour of parathyroid hormone- (PTH-) like hormone. The bowel can also rarely be affected by autoantibodies to myenteric neurones in association with small-cell carcinoma of the lung. In this situation, intestinal pseudo-obstruction develops. While severe constipation does occur with pseudo-obstruction, the main presentation is with small-bowel obstruction (leading to distension and vomiting).

5. DIARRHOEA

1. **C – Bacterial enterocolitis**
This patient has bacterial enterocolitis, as evidenced by the history of foreign travel and the symptoms and signs. A preceding flu-like 'prodrome' is also common before diarrhoea ensues. Common causative infective agents include *Escherichia coli* and species of *Salmonella*, *Shigella* and *Campylobacter*. Amoebic dysentery is by definition associated with bloody diarrhoea.

2. **D – Caecal carcinoma**
This gentleman has the classic clinical presentation of a caecal carcinoma, with a change in bowel habit (usually to diarrhoea), weight loss and microcytic anaemia.

3. **J – Ulcerative colitis**

This woman has ulcerative colitis, as evidenced by the history, clinical and haematological findings. While an infective cause cannot be absolutely excluded without stool culture (and this should be performed as a first-line investigation and certainly before steroids are considered), ulcerative colitis is the most common diagnosis in such a patient presenting in the UK. Crohn's disease is a less common cause of colitis (it usually presents with small-bowel disease).

4. **F – Irritable bowel syndrome**

This should be considered to be a diagnosis of exclusion and investigations should be performed (as in this case) to rule out an anatomical cause, particularly Crohn's disease. The disorder is then defined on the basis of the pattern of symptoms (using the Rome II criteria for functional bowel disorders). The pattern of alternating symptoms (constipation and diarrhoea) is characteristic, although either constipation or diarrhoea can predominate.

5. **H – Pseudomembranous colitis**

This is caused by overgrowth of *Clostridium difficile* after treatment with oral or intravenous broad-spectrum antibiotics. The diagnosis is confirmed by stool culture. Treatment involves stopping the causative agents and starting vancomycin. The disorder takes its name from the pseudomembrane that is observed if the colonic mucosa is examined endoscopically. In an 80–year-old, overflow diarrhoea and incontinence caused by faecal impaction should be excluded by rectal examination, as in this case.

6. WEIGHT LOSS

1. **H – Thyrotoxicosis**

This young woman has signs and symptoms consistent with thyrotoxicosis. The hypopigmentation is vitiligo, which is associated with several autoimmune disorders. Patients can have signs of Graves' disease, with the classic triad of acropachy (pseudo-clubbing) of the nails, Graves' orbitopathy (eye disease) and pre tibial myxoedema. Patients need to be started on carbimazole or propylthiouracil and might require some nutritional supplementation. Autoantibodies should be checked, including those associated with pernicious anaemia.

2. **J – Type 1 diabetes mellitus**

This teenager has developed type 1 diabetes mellitus. He requires a full examination, including screening for retinopathy, nephropathy and neuropathy. He will need education from a nurse specialist and will have to be started on insulin therapy. He will need review by a dietician and nutritional supplementation until he regains the weight he has lost.

3. **A – Alcohol dependency**

This woman has become depressed after her divorce and is now drinking excessive amounts of alcohol, as evidenced by her macrocytic anaemia, low urea and sodium, and deranged liver function tests (LFTs) and INR. She needs counselling and perhaps review by a psychiatrist. She should be given vitamin supplements, including daily thiamine.

4. **C – Carcinomatosis**

This woman has signs of disseminated malignancy, with ascites, hepatomegaly and multiple pulmonary metastases. The most likely cause is an ovarian cancer, which often presents late with evidence of intra-abdominal metastases. The diagnosis can be confirmed by ultrasound of the pelvis and/or an ascitic tap, which might show evidence of malignant cells.

5. **F – Crohn's disease**

This young man has returned from Nepal with a history suggestive of an acute infective diarrhoeal illness. The negative stool cultures and microscopy do not rule out an infective cause but make it less likely. The endoscopic findings and biopsy results, however, suggest that this is in fact his first presentation of Crohn's disease. The patient requires steroids, nutritional supplementation and education regarding his diagnosis.

7. ABDOMINAL PAIN I

1. **C – Ascending cholangitis**

This man has ascending cholangitis with the classic Charcot's triad of fever, rigors and jaundice. The low blood pressure is common in this disorder because of the effect of endotoxaemic shock caused by the Gram-negative organisms (mainly *Escherichia coli*) that cause this condition. This shock should be corrected and the sepsis treated aggressively because this condition carries a 30% mortality. A plain abdominal film might confirm the diagnosis (showing gas in the biliary tree). The commonest cause is gallstones.

2. **B – Appendicitis**

This patient has appendicitis, as evidenced by the short history of right iliac fossa pain and associated gastrointestinal upset with a leucocytosis. The diagnosis is a clinical one and one would also expect to find evidence of peritonism (guarding, rebound tenderness) in the right iliac fossa. Other causes of an identical picture could include Crohn's ileitis, but this is uncommon if there is no preceding history of abdominal symptoms.

3. **A – Acute pancreatitis**

This patient has acute pancreatitis, as evidenced by the history of alcohol abuse and the clinical presentation. The results confirm the dehydration and hypokalaemia associated with the prolonged vomiting, which is a marked feature of this abdominal condition. The raised WCC occurs secondary to pancreatic inflammation but might also indicate impending septic complications.

4. **E – Diverticulitis**

This patient has diverticulitis. This is very common for a woman of her age. The long previous history of pain and change in bowel habit is indicative of diverticulosis, and this has become complicated by inflammation in a diverticulum, leading to the increase in symptoms and peritonism in the left iliac fossa.

5. **J – Ureteric colic**

This patient has ureteric colic, which is caused by a calculus obstructing the right ureter. The appearance of a patient unable to get comfortable in any position is classic of this condition, which causes acute, very severe colicky pain that can be felt in the abdomen or loin and classically radiates to the groin or even to the tip of the penis. The finding of blood in the urine in a man invariably indicates pathology and is consistent with this diagnosis. The radiograph is normal because a proportion of ureteric stones are radiolucent. The confirmatory investigation would be an intravenous urogram (IVU), provided this is not contraindicated (asthma).

8. ABDOMINAL PAIN II

1. **D – Myocardial infarction**
This patient has had a myocardial infarction, as evidenced by the clinical findings and the raised cardiac enzymes (troponin and creatinine kinase). Inferior cardiac ischaemia commonly manifests as upper abdominal or epigastric pain and this should always be considered in the differential diagnosis.

2. **J – Small-bowel obstruction**
This patient has small-bowel obstruction, as evidenced by the symptoms of colicky central abdominal pain, vomiting and distension. She does not complain of absolute constipation, which is the fourth cardinal symptom of intestinal obstruction, because this occurs late in the time course of proximal bowel obstruction (see scenario 4). The commonest cause of small-intestinal obstruction in the Western world is adhesions (60% of patients). In this case, the likely cause of such adhesions is given – the previous intraperitoneal inflammation and surgery. The other common cause is a hernia.

3. **H – Ruptured abdominal aortic aneurysm**
This man has a ruptured abdominal aortic aneurysm, as evidenced by the sudden onset of severe pain associated with profound shock and generalised peritonism. In addition, he has the less constant finding of weak femoral pulses. Hypertension is the principal risk factor for aortic aneurysms in the Western world. More detailed history-taking, when possible, might elicit a long history of aching pain in the epigastrium or backache, which are both symptoms of aortic aneurysms. This is a surgical emergency and the immediate management includes oxygen administration and aggressive intravenous fluid/blood replacement.

4. **C – Large-bowel obstruction**
This woman has large-bowel obstruction, as evidenced by lower abdominal colic, distension and absolute constipation (failure to pass stool or flatus). Vomiting occurs late in large-bowel obstruction, in contrast to small-bowel obstruction when it is an early feature (see scenario 2). Tenderness should not be present in simple obstruction and is a sign of complications (ie ischaemia/perforation due to strangulation). The three most common causes of large-bowel obstruction in adulthood (in the developed world) are colorectal cancer, colonic volvulus and inflammatory stricture (especially secondary to diverticular disease).

5. **G – Perforated duodenal ulcer**
This man has a perforated duodenal ulcer, as evidenced by the characteristic rapid onset of severe, constant epigastric pain and the clinical finding of a rigid abdomen, which is indicative of generalised peritonitis (in this case chemical peritonitis from gastric acid). A silent abdomen, tachycardia and tachypnoea with shallow breathing

167

are invariable clinical features. This is another surgical emergency that is an indication for emergency laparotomy (usually with oversewing of the ulcer) after attention has been paid to fluid and electrolyte replacement.

9. ABDOMINAL MASS

1. **I – Pancreatic pseudocyst**
   This patient has a pancreatic pseudocyst. This is a collection of pancreatic secretions that collect in the lesser sac, and is caused by pancreatitis (it is one of the classic complications of pancreatitis). The patient might give a history of acute pancreatitis or might present with epigastric fullness, pain, nausea and, sometimes, vomiting. Such cysts can become complicated by infection or haemorrhage.

2. **B – Carcinoma of the head of the pancreas**
   This patient has a carcinoma of the head of the pancreas. The history and findings are of obstructive jaundice with a palpable gallbladder. Courvoisier's law states: 'When the gallbladder is palpable and the patient is jaundiced the obstruction of the bile duct causing the jaundice is unlikely to be a stone because previous inflammation will have made the gallbladder thick and non-distensible.' While there are a few exceptions to this rule, the history of substantial weight loss and of pain radiating to the left side of the back strongly indicate the likelihood of pancreatic carcinoma – the commonest cause of malignant biliary obstruction.

3. **D – Carcinoma of the sigmoid colon**
   This patient has a carcinoma of the sigmoid colon. The patient has presented with a late complication of the disease, ie extensive hepatic metastasis sufficient to obstruct biliary drainage. Colorectal cancer is the commonest cause of such intrahepatic obstruction. The patient therefore has two masses – the primary in the left iliac fossa and hepatomegaly.

4. **F – Cirrhosis of the liver**
   This patient has cirrhosis of the liver. She has presented with features of portal hypertension (decreased level of consciousness due to hepatic encephalopathy, ascites and haematemesis secondary to oesophageal varices). The liver is enlarged (the palpable mass) and she is jaundiced. Alcoholic liver cirrhosis is the commonest cause of jaundice and portal hypertension in the developed world.

5. **H – Gallstone disease**
   This patient has gallstone disease. This has become complicated by an empyema of the gallbladder. The gallbladder distension is caused by a stone obstructing the cystic duct, and the subsequent empyema (pus in the gallbladder) by infection of the stagnant bile. This mass is palpable in the right upper quadrant and associated with a systemic febrile illness. The patient is not jaundiced because the common bile duct and hepatic ducts are not obstructed.

10. DYSPHAGIA

1. **G – Oesophageal carcinoma**
    The history of rapidly progressive dysphagia in a man of this age should prompt this diagnosis. The weight loss and associated hypoproteinaemia are highly suggestive. A histological diagnosis would be confirmed by oesophagoscopy, and the size of the lesion estimated by barium swallow, which usually has a typical irregular, shouldered 'apple core' appearance.

2. **B – Bulbar palsy**
    Bulbar palsy is a palsy of the tongue, muscles of mastication, muscles of deglutition and facial muscles due to loss of function of brainstem motor nuclei. The signs are those of a lower motor neurone lesion. Bulbar palsy is one of the principal clinical patterns seen in motor neurone disease (25% of cases); other causes include Guillain–Barré syndrome, polio and brainstem tumours. Motor neurone disease never affects the extraocular movements, distinguishing it from myasthenia gravis. In contrast to bulbar palsy, pseudobulbar palsy is an upper motor neurone lesion.

3. **A – Achalasia**
    This is the commonest oesophageal motility disorder and is characterised by failure of relaxation of the lower oesophageal sphincter. Achalasia commonly presents between the ages of 30 and 60 with dysphagia for both solids and liquids equally, often with some associated pain. The cause is unclear. The diagnosis is confirmed by the characteristic beak-like tapering of the lower oesophagus on barium swallow. It can be confirmed by detailed measurements of pressures in the oesophageal lumen (manometry).

4. **F – Oesophageal candidiasis**
    This patient has oesophageal candidiasis, as evidenced by the short history of symptoms in a patient on immunosuppressive treatment. The disorder is also seen in patients with acquired immunodeficiency syndrome (AIDS), in which it can be the presenting symptom and can be a source of considerable morbidity.

5. **D – Gastro-oesophageal reflux disease (GORD)**
    This patient has gastro-oesophageal reflux disease (GORD), as evidenced by the long history of classic symptoms. The diagnosis is confirmed by the endoscopy, when he was found to have grade III disease (ie circumferential disease leading to a stricture). The pH study confirms increased lower oesophageal acid exposure (pH <4 for >4% of the time).

11. DISEASES OF THE STOMACH

1. **C – Adenocarcinoma**
    Epigastric pain is a non-specific symptom of upper gastrointestinal pathological conditions, but the weight loss and anorexia are more sinister, and the anaemia implies chronic gastrointestinal bleeding. The endoscopic appearance of a thickened, rigid gastric wall suggests linitis plastica (or 'leather bottle' stomach), a term used for gastric adenocarcinoma that diffusely infiltrates all layers of the gastric wall. The finding of numerous signet-ring cells on biopsy confirms a poorly differentiated (or diffuse) adenocarcinoma.

2. **B – Acute erosive gastritis**
This condition most commonly results from the ingestion of aspirin or non-steroidal anti-inflammatory drugs (NSAIDs), though alcohol excess, steroid therapy, chemotherapeutic agents and severe stress (such as from burns) can cause a similar picture. Endoscopically, the gastric mucosa is hyperaemic and shows partial-thickness mucosal defects (erosions). If the erosions bleed, melaena and/or anaemia can occur.

3. **I – Lymphoma of mucosa-associated lymphoid tissue (MALT)**
The normal gastric mucosa is virtually devoid of lymphocytes and any lymphocytic infiltrate in the stomach therefore signifies disease. The differential diagnosis of a heavy lymphocytic infiltrate lies between gastritis and lymphoma. In this patient, the facts that the lymphocytes are atypical and that there is intraepithelial involvement, coupled with the endoscopic appearance of thickened folds and ulceration suggest that the infiltrate is lymphomatous. MALT lymphomas are the most common type of primary gastric lymphoma and are usually of a low-grade B-cell type.

4. **H – Kaposi's sarcoma**
The endoscopic and histological features of this patient's gastric lesion are typical of Kaposi's sarcoma. This vascular tumour is the most common neoplasm found in patients with AIDS and, in contrast to HIV-negative patients (in whom it is virtually confined to the skin), it is often widely distributed and behaves aggressively. It has now been shown that Kaposi's sarcoma is caused by infection with a novel type of herpes virus known as human herpesvirus type 8.

5. **A – Active chronic gastritis**
In this patient, the lymphocytic infiltrate is due not to lymphoma, but to *Helicobacter pylori*-related chronic gastritis. Plasma cells and lymphoid follicles are commonly found throughout the mucosa in this type of gastritis. The presence of neutrophils indicates acute, or active inflammation and is also a feature of *H. pylori* gastritis. *H. pylori* is by far the most common cause of chronic gastritis worldwide, occurring in 80–90% of patients with antral gastritis.

6. **F – Chronic peptic ulcer**
The main differential diagnosis of a gastric ulcer lies between a chronic peptic ulcer and an ulcerating malignant tumour. Chronic peptic ulcers have sharply defined borders without any heaping-up of the epithelium surrounding the ulcer crater, in contrast to ulcerating malignancies which tend to have raised, rolled, everted edges. The floor of the peptic ulcer is composed of fibrous scar tissue overlaid by granulation tissue, inflammatory exudate and necrotic slough. The endoscopic and histological findings in this patient therefore support a diagnosis of chronic peptic ulcer. The mucosa adjacent to a chronic peptic ulcer often shows chronic gastritis, particularly when *Helicobacter pylori* infection is the underlying cause.

12. DYSPEPSIA AND PEPTIC ULCER DISEASE

1. **C – Duodenal ulcer**
This man has an obvious duodenal ulcer which is associated with a strongly positive CLO (*Campylobacter*-like organism) test, indicative of *Helicobacter pylori* infection. Approximately 90–95% of duodenal ulcers are associated with *H. pylori* infection and

often patients with a diagnosis of duodenal ulceration are treated empirically with anti-*H. pylori* therapy. Patients should be treated with 'triple therapy' for 1 week. This includes a proton-pump inhibitor and two antibiotics (eg lansoprazole, amoxicillin and metronidazole or omeprazole, amoxicillin and clarithromycin).

2.   **A – Barrett's oesophagus**
Barrett's oesophagus results from chronic gastro-oesophageal reflux disease and is a pre-malignant metaplasia of the epithelium. Patients with this condition need regular endoscopic monitoring and therapy with proton-pump inhibitors. Untreated, patients have a 30–40–fold increased risk of developing adenocarcinoma of the oesophagus.

3.   **I – Pyloric stenosis**
This patient has developed pyloric stenosis, as indicated by the projectile vomiting, the succussion splash and the hypokalaemic metabolic alkalosis. Other causes include congenital stenosis seen in babies, obstructing tumours of the pylorus, active peptic ulcers, scarred healed peptic ulcers, and external compression due to tumours. Patients require a surgical resection procudure to relieve the outflow tract obstruction.

4.   **H – Oesophageal stricture**
This patient has a history suggestive of oesophageal stricture. The level of the dysphagia should be ascertained, as should the nature of the dysphagia, ie what food consistency the patient can manage. Other important questions include the association of 'impact pain' that usually occurs with benign disease, and regurgitation of food, which might indicate absolute obstruction. Endoscopy or barium swallow is used to diagnose the lesion but biopsy is required to confirm whether the lesion is benign or malignant. Benign strictures are usually a result of reflux disease and require treatment with a proton-pump inhibitor and regular dilation. Malignant disease should be resecteds if appropriate.

5.   **J – Zollinger–Ellison syndrome**
This man has Zollinger–Ellison syndrome, multiple peptic ulcers caused by a gastrinoma, a rare tumour of the G-cells of the pancreas. Patients present with multiple peptic ulcers and diarrhoea due to the low pH in the upper bowel. Treatment includes proton-pump inhibitors, octreotide and, if possible, resection of the tumour.

13. TREATMENT OF DYSPEPSIA

1.   **G – Misoprostol**
Misoprostol is a synthetic prostaglandin analogue that is principally used as a prophylactic agent against NSAID-induced upper gastrointestinal ulceration. It commonly causes diarrhoea, particularly in the elderly, and this might require it to be stopped. It also causes upper gastrointestinal symptoms, including nausea and abdominal discomfort. It should not be given to women of childbearing age as it can cause menstrual irregularities and spontaneous abortion in pregnancy.

2.   **E – Cimetidine**
Cimetidine is an H_2-antagonist that works by blocking parietal-cell production and secretion of hydrochloric acid. Cimetidine causes nausea, diarrhoea and, in long-term use, gynaecomastia. Other causes of gynaecomastia include digoxin, spironolactone,

cannabis, heroin, cyproterone and oestrogens. Beware the dyspeptic hippie with atrial fibrillation, hypertension and carcinoma of the prostate!

3. **A – Aluminium hydroxide**

Antacid preparations can be bought over the counter (as can H_2-antagonists) and are commonly 'abused' by patients who self-medicate for their dyspepsia. They give good symptomatic relief but rarely effect healing of the cause of their dyspepsia. Aluminium-based medications cause constipation, while magnesium salts cause diarrhoea.

4. **C – Calcium carbonate**

This patient has a metabolic alkalosis, as evidenced by her raised serum bicarbonate and pH. Both calcium carbonate and carbenoxolone can cause this problem but carbenoxolone (a liquorice derivative) is not available over the counter. It is reserved for patients with poorly responsive peptic ulceration.

5. **B – Bismuth**

This patient has been placed on bismuth chelate, as part of a second-line triple therapy. Bismuth has a direct anti-*Helicobacter pylori* effect, coating the ulcer surface and protecting it against the direct effects of the intraluminal acid. It is reserved for patients with poorly responsive ulceration.

14. MALABSORPTION

1. **I – Tuberculous terminal ileitis**

This man has developed terminal ileitis secondary to tuberculosis. A similar picture can develop secondary to Crohn's disease and 'backwash ileitis' due to proximal ulcerative colitis. Inflammatory bowel disease is uncommon in Asian and South-East Asian populations and tuberculosis should always be excluded in such cases. Patients require anti-tuberculous therapy for 6–12 months and vitamin supplementation, particularly vitamin B_{12} (which is absorbed in the distal ileum).

2. **D – Coeliac disease**

This young woman has developed coeliac disease (gluten-sensitive enteropathy). Patients most commonly present with non-specific changes in bowel habit and it is unusual to have frank steatorrhoea. Mouth ulceration and weight loss are also common, as is anaemia, which is due to iron or folate deficiency. The diagnosis is confirmed by the presence of anti-endomysial and anti-tissue transglutaminase antibodies, and by the appearance of subtotal villous atrophy on small-bowel biopsies (taken endoscopically). Patients should be treated with nutritional supplements and a gluten-free diet. People with coeliac disease have an increased risk of all upper gastrointestinal malignancies, in particular small-bowel lymphoma.

3. **B – Bacterial overgrowth**

Altered anatomy due to bowel resection, fistulae or strictures can lead to bacterial overgrowth in the small bowel and subsequent malabsorption. The diagnosis can be confirmed by blood tests, including a full blood count (which will show a macrocytic anaemia secondary to vitamin B_{12} deficiency); serum folate, which might be raised due to the bacterial production and subsequent absorption of tetrahydrofolate; urea and electrolytes (U&Es); LFTs (hypoalbuminaemia); and deconjugated bile acids (raised).

Faecal fat and Schilling tests might be helpful but the ^{14}C breath test is diagnostic. There are two forms of the test, ^{14}C-xylose and ^{14}C-cholyglycine. The first is based on the labelled xylose being metabolised by Gram-negative aerobic organisms to $^{14}CO_2$ and xylose. The carbon dioxide is subsequently absorbed in the small bowel and excreted via the breath. The other test relies on anaerobic organisms deconjugating the labelled bile acid to ^{14}C-glycine. This is absorbed and metabolised in the liver, releasing $^{14}CO_2$, which is excreted via the breath.

4. J – Tropical sprue

Tropical sprue is a diagnosis of exclusion that has been defined as 'malabsorption occurring in defined areas of the tropics in which no bacterial, viral or parasitic infection can be detected'. In fact, the diagnosis should only be considered when all other causes of malabsorption have been excluded, including infective, infiltrative, malignant and metabolic causes. The aetiology of this disorder is thought to be infective but the actual cause and pathology remains unclear. The disorder is restricted to definite endemic areas around the tropics and it can occur in epidemics in indigenous populations. Travellers can suffer with the condition after an initial acute diarrhoeal illness but this does not necessarily happen in all cases. Patients returning to a Western diet and environment might have spontaneous resolution of their symptoms but some people require nutritional support (particularly vitamin B_{12} and folate) and a course of tetracycline. The use of antibiotics is still of unproved benefit.

5. C – Chronic pancreatitis

This man has evidence of chronic pancreatitis, chronic liver disease and malabsorption. He has a macrocytic anaemia (vitamin B_{12} and folate deficiencies and alcohol excess), thrombocytopenia, hyponatraemia and deranged LFTs (alcohol excess) and hypoalbuminaemia (alcohol and malabsorption). He also has evidence of hyperglycaemia secondary to pancreatic insufficiency and the abdominal radiograph shows calcification in the upper abdomen, characteristic of chronic pancreatitis. He should be encouraged to refrain from alcohol and he needs treatment for his diabetes, malabsorption and nutritional deficiencies. He will require insulin and pancreatic enzyme replacement.

15. INFECTIVE DIARRHOEA

1. C – *Clostridium difficile*

Clostridium difficile is one of the principal organisms associated with antibiotic-induced diarrhoea. It is carried by 3–5% of the normal population as part of their gut flora but can be spread in hospitals through poor hygiene. Broad-spectrum antibiotics render the individual susceptible to infection but can also cause overgrowth. It carries a high mortality in the elderly and requires prompt recognition, isolation and treatment. Its pathogenicity is due to two toxins, an enterotoxin, responsible for the diarrhoea, and a cytotoxin, responsible for the 'pseudomembrane', which is almost pathognomonic. Treatment includes maintenance of hydration and oral metronidazole or vancomycin.

2. A – *Bacillus cereus*

Bacillus cereus is a common pathogen associated with food poisoning, particularly due to poorly reheated rice. Symptoms can start 1–2 hours after ingestion of affected food materials, but can be delayed by as much as 8–16 hours. Its pathogenicity is due to an enterotoxin but it is usually a self-limiting condition and patients require only supportive fluid replacement.

3. **F – *Giardia lamblia***
    Giardia lamblia is a common pathogen with a worldwide distribution. It is commonly found in Eastern Europe and Russia and causes both malabsorption and watery diarrhoea. It characteristically causes foul-smelling flatus! Initially the organism colonises and multiplies in the small bowel, causing partial villous atrophy and malabsorption. As it passes into the large bowel it causes watery diarrhoea. Like amoebae, this flagellate organism can exist in cyst and trophozoite forms, which can be found in the stool. Specific antibodies can also be detected in the serum, including an acute-phase IgM response. Treatment includes rehydration and oral metronidazole.

4. **J – *Vibrio cholerae***
    Vibrio cholerae is a Gram-negative bacillus that is responsible for epidemic and pandemic outbreaks of diarrhoea, particularly in developing-world areas. Two varieties of the disease may occur. The more common severe illness starts 1–5 days after infection. Initially there is profuse watery diarrhoea, which classically takes on a 'rice water' appearance due to flecks of mucus within the fluid. This marks the beginning of a severe diarrhoeal illness, with vomiting, dehydration and cardiovascular collapse soon intervening. Without rehydration therapy and tetracycline patients will soon die. More unusually the disease can manifest as a milder illness. In epidemics the main problem is identifying asymptomatic carriers and maintaining adequate sanitation to stop the spread of the disease. In recent years drug resistance has become an increasing problem.

5. **D – *Cryptosporidium***
    Cryptosporidium usually causes a mild, self-limiting diarrhoeal illness that can last for up to 10 days. However, in immunocompromised patients it can cause a severe diarrhoeal illness associated with toxic dilatation of the colon. Treatment includes hydration, nutritional and electrolyte support. Despite numerous trials, there does not as yet appear to be an effective therapy for this infection in HIV patients.

16. TYPES OF COLITIS

1. **L – Ulcerative colitis**
    The main differential diagnosis of bloody diarrhoea in this age group lies between infective colitis and idiopathic inflammatory bowel disease. The fact that repeated stool cultures are negative makes infective colitis less likely. The colonoscopic appearances of diffuse erythema without skip lesions favour ulcerative colitis over Crohn's disease. The biopsy changes (severe chronic inflammation limited to the mucosa, with crypt abscesses and crypt architectural distortion) are typical of ulcerative colitis.

2. **H – Ischaemic colitis**
    In an elderly patient with bloody diarrhoea, ischaemic colitis should be added to the differential diagnosis list, particularly in a patient known to have arterial disease. Partial or complete occlusion of the inferior mesenteric artery is a recognised complication of reconstructive arterial surgery, resulting in hypoperfusion of the distal large intestine. The most susceptible areas are the splenic flexure and rectum, both of which are watershed

zones. Ulceration and haemorrhage are seen in the early stages with progression to infarction in severe cases. Stricture formation can occur as a consequence of healing.

3.   D – Crohn's colitis
The only granulomatous disease on this list is Crohn's disease. Growth failure is a common consequence of this disease in children, in addition to the symptoms of abdominal pain and diarrhoea. The colonoscopic findings of so-called 'skip lesions', with the affected areas showing linear ulceration, is typical of Crohn's disease.

4.   J – Pseudomembranous colitis
Pseudomembranous colitis is caused by the A and B toxins produced by toxigenic strains of *Clostridium difficile*. It usually occurs a few days after starting broad-spectrum antibiotic therapy and most commonly affects elderly, hospitalised patients. Diarrhoea (rarely with blood) and abdominal cramps are the common symptoms. Sigmoidoscopy might reveal an erythematous, ulcerated mucosa with patchy white membranes. In a minority of patients, however, only the proximal colon is affected and sigmoidoscopy is therefore normal.

5.   C – Collagenous colitis
In some patients with diarrhoea the large intestine is normal at colonoscopy but inflammation is detected histologically on biopsies. In this situation, a diagnosis of 'microscopic colitis' is made. This is not a specific diagnosis, however, but an umbrella term covering several conditions. One of these conditions is collagenous colitis. This disease occurs most commonly in middle-aged women, who develop profuse watery diarrhoea. The colonoscopy is normal but the colonic biopsies show mucosal inflammation and a thick subepithelial band of collagen.

6.   G – Infective colitis
Certain bacterial infections of the colon cause a colitis that mimics idiopathic inflammatory bowel disease. The most important pathogens in this group are *Salmonella* species, *Shigella* species, enteroinvasive *Escherichia coli* and *Campylobacter* species. Typically, all these organisms produce similar symptoms, namely abdominal pain and diarrhoea, often with blood. The sigmoidoscopic appearances of diffuse mucosal erythema with ulceration are also similar, irrespective of the pathogen, and can be mistaken for ulcerative colitis. The typical biopsy findings are acute inflammation and oedema.

17. INFLAMMATORY BOWEL DISEASE

1.   J – Sclerosing cholangitis
The blood results of this patient suggest a cholestatic jaundice, with a relatively raised alkaline phosphatase compared with the transaminases and bilirubin. The endoscopic retrograde cholangiopancreatiogram (ERCP) shows the characteristic 'beading', which represents alternating areas of strictures and dilatations. Patients usually present with jaundice and cholangitis but can be asymptomatic or present with cirrhosis. The disorder is principally associated with ulcerative colitis (rarely occurring with Crohn's disease) and is unrelated to the activity of the colitis.

2. **G – Oxalate renal stones**
    This patient has developed renal oxalate stones as a result of his multiple small-bowel resections. Oxalate is normally bound to calcium in the terminal ileum, rendering it insoluble and so non-absorbable in the colon. In patients who have had small-bowel resection this cannot occur and oxalate is absorbed in the colon, leading to hyperoxaluria and subsequent stone formation.

3. **A – Anterior uveitis**
    This patient has presented with anterior uveitis and symptoms of colitis. Anterior uveitis is usually related to the disease activity and can be an associated presenting symptom, as in this case. Anterior uveitis has a similar incidence (4–5%) in both ulcerative colitis and Crohn's disease.

4. **H – Pyoderma gangrenosum**
    Pyoderma gangrenosum occurs more commonly with ulcerative colitis and is usually related to the disease activity. The lesion can be seen in inflammatory bowel disease, vasculitic disorders and haematological malignancies.

5. **F – Gallstones**
    Gallstones are a common finding in patients with inflammatory bowel disease, occurring with a several-fold increased incidence in patients with Crohn's disease but with a normal incidence in patients with ulcerative colitis. The diagnosis can be confirmed by ultrasound scan and ERCP. Stones in the common bile duct can be removed at ERCP and stenting of the duct might be required to prevent further obstruction.

18. RECTAL BLEEDING

1. **C – Colonic carcinoma**
    This patient has a colonic carcinoma, as evidenced by the history of a change in bowel habit and weight loss in an elderly man with dark-red rectal bleeding. The full blood count shows anaemia of chronic disease, which is typical for such a patient.

2. **J – Ulcerative colitis**
    This patient has ulcerative colitis. This is the commonest diagnosis in a young patient with a long history of bloody diarrhoea. The microcytic anaemia reflects chronic blood loss, and the white cell count (WCC) and erythrocyte sedimentation rate (ESR) reflect the underlying inflammatory condition.

3. **D – Colonic polyp**
    This man has a colonic polyp. A history of fresh bleeding in the absence of any other symptoms or findings on examination suggests this diagnosis in a man of this age, although a small carcinoma cannot be excluded.

4. **G – Haemorrhoids**
    This man has haemorrhoids. Bright-red rectal bleeding in a young patient without any other abdominal symptoms probably has a local anal cause and a fissure is unlikely without pain on defecation. It is very uncommon to find anaemia in patients who only have haemorrhoidal bleeding.

5. **H – Infective colitis**
    This young woman has infective colitis. This is suggested by the foreign travel where such disorders are commonplace and the short history of abdominal pain and bloody diarrhoea (dysentery). The two commonest organisms implicated are *Shigella* spp. (bacterial dysentery) and *Entamoeba histolytica* (amoebic dysentery). Infections arise from faecally contaminated water supplies.

19. ANORECTAL CONDITIONS

1. **F – Haemorrhoids**
    This patient has haemorrhoids. His symptoms are bleeding and the sensation of the haemorrhoids protruding through the anal canal. These require digital replacement, so he has third-degree haemorrhoids. The differential diagnosis could include a prolapsing rectal polyp.

2. **A – Anal carcinoma**
    This patient has an anal carcinoma, as evidenced by the history and findings on examination. This must always be excluded in a patient presenting with any anal symptoms in this age group and a biopsy should therefore be taken. Similarly, when ulceration or fissuring is not situated posteriorly or anteriorly (ie at the 12-o'clock or 6-o'clock positions) this diagnosis should be considered in a patient of any age.

3. **J – Rectal prolapse**
    This patient has a full-thickness rectal prolapse. This is a common cause of faecal incontinence in the elderly. The full thickness of the rectum and lower part of the anal canal evert, appearing as a long tubular mass protruding symmetrically through the anus. The exposed mucosa is red and is thrown into concentric folds around a central pit which is the lumen.

4. **C – Anal fistula**
    This patient has an anal fistula. The diagnosis is suggested by the symptoms of watery or purulent discharge causing excoriation of the perianal skin and pruritus ani, and the finding of puckered scarring on examination. In addition, however, the abdominal symptoms are strongly suggestive of Crohn's disease which is the cause in about 50% of all fistulae.

5. **H – Perianal haematoma**
    This patient has a perianal haematoma, as evidenced by the short history and clinical findings of a painful subcutaneous lump at the anal verge. A perianal haematoma is not a haemorrhoidal complication. They are caused instead by a rupture or acute thrombosis of one of the small veins of the subcutaneous perianal plexus.

20. COMMON ABDOMINAL OPERATIONS

1.   **E – Hartmann's procedure**
     This patient has had a Hartmann's procedure, as indicated by the cause for surgery, and the finding of an end-colostomy. This procedure is usually performed as an emergency for inflammatory or obstructing conditions affecting the sigmoid region of the colon (especially in high-risk patients). The diseased or obstructed area is excised, but an anastomosis of the bowel is not undertaken for safety reasons at the time of surgery, and because of a high risk of anastomotic dehiscence post-operatively. The proximal colon is therefore brought to the skin as the stoma, and the rectal stump is oversewn. The colostomy can be reversed at a later date, but this in itself is no small undertaking.

2.   **J – Right hemicolectomy**
     This patient has had a right hemicolectomy, as indicated by the cause for surgery. Crohn's disease predominantly affects the terminal ileum (ileitis) leading to stricturing and episodic small-bowel obstruction. The segment is commonly removed by right hemicolectomy, which removes the affected ileum and the proximal colon.

3.   **D – Emergency laparotomy**
     This patient has had an emergency laparotomy, as indicated by the cause for surgery. The term describes the opening of the abdomen in order to diagnose (and usually treat) a pathological abnormality, and might be performed for a variety of reasons, including trauma or perforated ulcer. The operation in itself would not make a good long case, but in combination with the hernia and his heart valve, it gives the examiner plenty of scope for entertainment. Remember, surgical patients make good long cases, and are therefore not uncommon!

4.   **I – Proctocolectomy with pouch ileoanal anastomosis (restorative proctocolectomy)**
     This patient has had a proctocolectomy with pouch ileoanal anastomosis (restorative proctocolectomy). This is indicated by the cause for surgery and by the description of her operations. The procedure is almost exclusively performed for ulcerative colitis and familial adenomatous polyposis, when the whole colon and rectum must be resected (because it is all affected by the disease process). The operation usually has two stages. The bowel is resected, with the formation of a neorectum from the distal ileum (the pouch) and primary anastomosis of this to the remaining anal canal. This operation is covered with a defunctioning loop ileostomy, which is later closed (the second operation).

5.   **A – Abdominoperineal excision of the rectum (APER)**
     This patient has had an abdominoperineal excision of the rectum (APER), as indicated by the cause for surgery and the fact that the rectum and anus have been completely excised, leaving a permanent colostomy and no anus. The operation is predominantly performed for very low rectal tumours that are too low for removal by anterior resection of the rectum.

21. ANATOMY OF THE INGUINAL REGION

1. E – Indirect inguinal hernia

The hernia passes along the spermatic cord from the deep inguinal ring. The neck of the sac is therefore lateral to the inferior epigastric vessels, which run directly upwards from the femoral artery at the mid-inguinal point.

2. D – Femoral hernia

The femoral ring is bordered laterally by the femoral vein and medially by the crescentic edge of the lacunar ligament. Anteriorly lies the medial part of the inguinal ligament and posteriorly the pectineal ligament.

3. H – Mid-point of the inguinal ligament

The deep inguinal ring lies just above the mid-point of the inguinal ligament. This should not be confused with the mid-inguinal point, which lies midway between the symphysis pubis and the anterior superior iliac spine and marks the site of the femoral artery as it passes under the inguinal ligament.

4. C – External oblique

The external oblique muscle covers the inguinal canal and must be incised in the line of its fibres to reveal the contents of the inguinal canal. Its diverging fibres at the medial end form the superficial inguinal ring.

5. J – Transversalis fascia

There are three coverings of the cord derived from each layer through which it passes on leaving the peritoneal cavity: the internal spermatic fascia (from the transversalis fascia), the cremasteric fascia (from the transversus abdominis and internal oblique muscles) and the external spermatic fascia (from the external oblique muscle).

22. HERNIAS

1. I – Strangulated hernia

The clinical findings are those of strangulation, which occurs when the blood supply to the contents of a hernia is cut off by tight constriction of the neck of the hernial sac. When a loop of gut is strangulated, there is also intestinal obstruction, as in this case. These patients are often very sick and require intensive preoperative resuscitation before hernia repair, which often necessitates small-bowel resection.

2. H – Spigelian hernia

This is the clinical and anatomical description of a Spigelian hernia. In contrast to common hernias (ie inguinal, femoral, para-umbilical, incisional and epigastric), this is one of the rarer types of hernia. Other rare hernias include lumbar, gluteal and obturator hernias.

3. G – Sliding hernia

The patient has a sliding hernia. The bowel, which is usually extraperitoneal, forms one side of the sac, and has slid down the canal, pulling peritoneum with it (hence the name). The sac can contain other loops of bowel. The most common site is a left inguinal hernia, where the extraperitoneal component is the sigmoid colon. While complications such as strangulation can occur, the common problem with these hernias is surgical error, as in this case.

4. **A – Incarcerated hernia**
    The contents are fixed in the sac because of their size or adhesions. The hernia is irreducible but the bowel is not strangulated or obstructed. This patient has an incarcerated para-umbilical hernia, which is a common hernia through a defect that is adjacent to the umbilicus; the content is usually extraperitoneal fat/omentum. True umbilical hernias (ie those through the centre of the umbilicus) can be congenital (infants) or acquired. The acquired form is much less common than para-umbilical hernias and are invariably due to increased intra-abdominal pressure. They therefore occur with pregnancy, with ascites and with some other causes of marked abdominal distension.

5. **D – Obstructed hernia**
    This patient has the three cardinal symptoms of obstruction. Remember, adhesions and hernias are the two commonest causes of small-bowel obstruction in adults. Unlike strangulated hernias, the sac itself is not tender. Such patients require operative intervention, but are not generally as unwell as those with strangulation.

23. ANATOMY OF THE LIVER

1. **H – Quadrate lobe**
    The quadrate lobe is part of the right lobe of the liver, lying adjacent to the interlobar fissure. It is limited superiorly by the porta hepatis and protrudes onto the anterior surface between the fundus of the gallbladder and the falciform ligament.

2. **G – Porta hepatis**
    The free margin of the lesser sac contains the portal vein, hepatic artery and the common bile duct. These enter the liver at the porta hepatis. This transverse fissure forms the crosspiece of the H-shaped markings on the posterior liver surface. The vertical line on the left side is the interlobar fissure, and on the right, the inferior vena cava and the gallbladder. The caudate lobe lies above the porta hepatis within the lesser sac and the quadrate lobe below.

3. **C – Coronary ligament**
    The upper and lower layers of the coronary ligament enclose the bare area of the posterior surface of the right lobe. The layers meet laterally to form the right triangular ligament. The area has no peritoneal coverings and is in contact with the diaphragm, the inferior vena cava, and the right adrenal gland, overlying the upper pole of the right kidney.

4. **E – Left lobe**
    The right and left lobes are divided posteriorly by the vertical interlobar fissure containing the ligamentum venosus above, and the ligamentum teres below. Anteriorly, the line of demarcation is that of the falciform ligament, joining the superior and anterior surfaces of the liver to the diaphragm and anterior abdominal wall. The left lobe is attached posteriorly to the diaphragm by the left triangular ligament. It is related posteriorly to the oesophagus, the fundus of the stomach and the lesser omentum, the latter separating it from the pancreas.

5.   **B – Caudate process**
A finger passed into the lesser sac through its opening (the foramen of Winslow, aditus) passes behind the free margin of the lesser omentum, with the caudate process above and the first part of the duodenum below. The finger lies anterior to the peritoneum covering the inferior vena cava. The caudate process leads to the caudate lobe between the interlobar fissure and the lower layer of the coronary ligament. The lobe lies within, and at the apex of the lesser sac.

24. JAUNDICE

1.   **F – Gilbert's syndrome**
This man has Gilbert's syndrome, a relatively common cause of an unconjugated hyperbilirubinaemia associated with acute illness. The disorder is thought to be inherited in an autosomal dominant manner but maight have several modes of inheritance. It has a prevalence of 1–2% in the UK population. Patients present with an acute illness which is associated with a raised bilirubin. There are no other signs of derangement in the liver function tests and it is rare that patients present with frank jaundice, although they can have icteric sclerae.

2.   **G – Hepatitis A infection**
This man has developed an acute viral hepatitis as a result of hepatitis A virus infection. This is an RNA virus which is spread by the faecal–oral route. It causes an acute illness which can be associated with jaundice, diarrhoea and fever. In the acute phase, an anti-hepatitis A virus IgM response is seen and later an anti-hepatitis A virus IgG response confirms previous exposure and immunity. There is no chronic phase or associated carrier state with this infection, although, rarely, the acute infection can develop into fulminant liver failure.

3.   **B – Budd–Chiari syndrome**
This patient has developed hepatic vein obstruction secondary to thrombosis as a result of her polycythaemia rubra vera. This disorder is known as the 'Budd–Chiari syndrome' and in the majority of cases it arises secondary to thrombogenic disorders, including myeloproliferative disorders, protein C, protein S, factor V Leiden, and antithrombin III deficiencies, the oral contraceptive pill and pregnancy. Rarely it can be due to a congenital web within the hepatic vein. The diagnosis can be confirmed by ultrasound scan and venography of the hepatic vein and inferior vena cava (which are involved in up to 20% of cases). Treatment includes anticoagulation and treatment of the underlying cause.

4.   **J – Primary biliary cirrhosis**
This middle-aged woman has signs of a chronic liver disease associated with acute jaundice. The autoantibodies are highly suggestive of primary biliary cirrhosis. The disease is often heralded by the onset of pruritus, which can occur several months before any of the other features are manifest. It is characterised immunologically by the presence of the antimitochondrial antibody. Anti-smooth muscle antibodies (principally associated with autoimmune hepatitis) can also be present. Patients should have a liver biopsy to determine the stage and prognosis of the condition. Progression of the disease is variable but few of the current therapies have been shown to greatly influence it. Prognostic markers include serum albumin, bilirubin, prothrombin time

and evidence of cirrhosis and portal hypertension. Liver transplantation might be considered in some cases.

5. **C – Carcinoma of the head of pancreas**
    This man has presented with symptoms suggestive of an obstructive jaundice. Painless jaundice in this age group should be considered to be secondary to carcinoma of the head of the pancreas until proved otherwise. Other causes can include cholangiocarcinoma, hepatic tumours and, rarely, obstructing tumours at the ampulla of Vater. The diagnosis can be confirmed on ultrasonography can but is usually made by ERCP and/or CT of the abdomen.

25. DISEASES OF THE LIVER

1. **H – Primary biliary cirrhosis**
    The clinical features of pruritus and jaundice and the raised alkaline phosphatase are strongly suggestive of biliary obstruction. The autoantibody profile is characteristic of primary biliary cirrhosis. The other abnormalities, namely the raised IgM and cholesterol and the granulomatous inflammation on liver biopsy, while not in themselves specific, support the diagnosis. Primary biliary cirrhosis is a chronic disorder in which there is progressive destruction of bile ducts, eventually leading to cirrhosis. Around 90% of affected patients are women aged 40–50. The disease is autoimmune in origin and is associated with other autoimmune disorders such as Sjögren's syndrome and rheumatoid arthritis.

2. **E – Chronic hepatitis B**
    The differential diagnosis of this viral hepatitis lies between chronic hepatitis B and hepatitis C. The fact that the infecting virus is a double-stranded DNA virus indicates that it is hepatitis B. Chronic hepatitis B is often not preceded by an acute hepatitic illness and patients are commonly asymptomatic. The severity of the disease at presentation varies from mild hepatitis to full-blown cirrhosis; 50% of patients have established chronic disease. Hepatitis B leads to liver cell damage, not via a cytopathic effect but by causing expression of viral antigens on the cell surface (HBsAg). The infected cells are recognised by the body's immune system and destroyed. If immunity is impaired, the virus can survive in the liver cells without causing damage and the patient becomes a chronic carrier. HbsAg can be detected in liver cell cytoplasm by specific immunohistochemical stains.

3. **F – Genetic haemochromatosis**
    Genetic (or primary) haemochromatosis is due to a gene defect on chromosome 6, near the HLA-A locus. The defect causes excessive absorption of iron in the small intestine. For many years the iron is deposited as haemosiderin in hepatocytes without any clinical effects. Eventually, however, the iron deposition becomes more extensive, involving Kupffer cells, bile duct epithelium and portal tract connective tissue. This causes hepatic fibrosis, followed by cirrhosis. Haemosiderin is also deposited in other organs such as the pancreas and heart, causing diabetes and cardiac failure. The discoloration of the skin is due to raised levels of melanotrophin.

4.   **D – Budd–Chiari syndrome**
In this patient the liver biopsy shows obstruction to the venous outflow of the liver. This is not a specific finding, but from the list given, the most likely cause is Budd–Chiari syndrome. This condition is due to occlusion of the hepatic vein and is most common in patients with hypercoagulable states, such as polycythaemia rubra vera, and in patients with posterior abdominal wall tumours that obstruct the hepatic vein. This patient's signs and symptoms, namely nausea, abdominal pain, hepatomegaly and ascites, are typical of the acute form of the disease. Magnetic resonance imaging (MRI) and Doppler ultrasound are useful investigations to confirm the hepatic vein occlusion.

5.   **J – Wilson's disease**
Wilson's disease is an inherited autosomal recessive disorder in which copper accumulates in the liver and in the basal ganglia of the brain. The underlying gene defect is on chromosome 13. This results in an abnormal copper-transporting ATPase and failure of the liver to excrete copper in the bile. In addition, there is a low serum caeruloplasmin in 80% of patients due to poor synthesis. Accumulation of copper in the liver causes chronic hepatitis and, eventually, cirrhosis. Copper deposition in the brain causes severe progressive neurological disability. Children usually present with hepatic problems while adults tend to present with neurological disease. A pathognomonic sign of Wilson's disease is the Kayser–Fleischer ring, which is due to copper deposition in the cornea.

26. DRUG-INDUCED JAUNDICE

1.   **J – Rifampicin**
This patient has been started on rifampicin for suspected *Legionella* pneumonia. Rifampicin is a hepatic enzyme inducer and can cause acute jaundice. It is commonly used for tuberculous infection and prophylaxis in meningococcal meningitis and patients need to be warned that their secretions will turn red, particularly urine and tears.

2.   **E – Erythromycin**
Erythromycin is commonly used as a substitute for penicillin when patients are known to be allergic to penicillin. Erythromycin is a hepatic enzyme inhibitor and must be used with caution when patients are on warfarin. It can cause a cholestatic jaundice.

3.   **A – Amiodarone**
Amiodarone is commonly used in the elderly to treat paroxysmal atrial fibrillation. Prior to starting patients on the drug they should be warned of the possible side-effects, which include: photosensitivity; a slate-grey discoloration of the skin; derangement of thyroid function, leading to biochemical and clinical dysthyroid disease; derangement of the liver function tests, causing jaundice, hepatitis and cirrhosis; reversible micro-corneal deposits; and pulmonary fibrosis.

4.   **G – Lisinopril**
This patient describes the classic dry, irritating 'ACE inhibitor cough'. The angiotensin-converting enzyme (ACE) inhibitors can cause derangement of the LFTs, hepatitis and a cholestatic jaundice, as evidenced in this case by the relatively raised alkaline phosphatase compared with the transaminases and bilirubin. It is usually reversible and resolves with cessation of the drug.

5. **B – Azathioprine**
    Azathioprine is a disease-modifying agent used as a third-line therapy in rheumatoid arthritis. It is also used in transplant patients and in inflammatory bowel disease. Its main side-effect is marrow suppression but it also causes hepatotoxicity, in particular cholestatic jaundice. Treatment should be monitored with regular full blood counts and liver function tests.

27. ASCITES

1. **I – Ovarian carcinoma**
    The two malignant tumours in the list are ovarian carcinoma and malignant mesothelioma, and the differential diagnosis therefore lies between these two. Distinguishing between them can sometimes be difficult on cytological examination of ascitic fluid but the fact that adenocarcinoma cells have been found indicates ovarian carcinoma.

2. **J – Tuberculosis**
    Tuberculosis is the archetypal granulomatous disease, and must always be considered in the differential diagnosis whenever granulomas are found. None of the other diseases in the list typically produce granulomas, although macrophages can be seen in ascitic fluid in many inflammatory conditions.

3. **H – Nephrotic syndrome**
    Nephrotic syndrome is characterised by heavy proteinuria, which leads to hypoalbuminaemia, peripheral oedema and ascites. In addition, nearly all patients have hyperlipidaemia with raised cholesterol, triglycerides and lipoproteins. The cause of the hyperlipidaemia is complex but is due in part to increased synthesis of lipoproteins in the liver, abnormal transport of lipid molecules and reduced catabolism. Lipiduria follows the hyperlipidaemia; the lipid is seen in the urine either as free fat or as oval fat bodies.

4. **B – Acute pancreatitis**
    The diagnosis of acute pancreatitis depends on measurement of the serum amylase. A raised serum amylase can be seen in other acute abdominal emergencies, such as perforated duodenal ulcer or intestinal infarction, but if the serum amylase is more than five times greater than normal, acute pancreatitis is highly likely.

5. **C – Alcoholic cirrhosis**
    Gamma-glutamyltransferase (γGT) is a microsomal enzyme that is found in the liver and in many other tissues. Its activity can be induced by drugs such as phenytoin and alcohol. When the alkaline phosphatase is normal, a raised serum γGT is a good guide to alcohol intake and can be used as a screening test. In the presence of cholestasis, however, the γGT rises in parallel with the alkaline phosphatase as it has a similar pathway of excretion.

28. DISORDERS OF THE PANCREAS

1. F – Gastrinoma

Most duodenal ulcers are solitary and located in the first part of the duodenum, so the distribution of ulcers in this patient (multiple ulcers throughout the second and third parts of the duodenum) is somewhat unusual. Intractable peptic ulcers, multiple ulcers or ulcers in uncommon sites are characteristic of Zollinger–Ellison syndrome. This is caused by excess secretion of gastrin from a gastrinoma. Gastrinomas are neuroendocrine tumours that are most often located in the pancreas, but are also found in other parts of the gastrointestinal tract, notably the duodenum. Despite their 'benign' name, many gastrinomas behave in a malignant fashion.

2. A – Acute haemorrhagic pancreatitis

Acute haemorrhagic pancreatitis typically presents with sudden onset of abdominal pain accompanied by signs of shock such as tachycardia, hypotension and tachypnoea. The two most common causes of acute pancreatitis are gallstones and alcohol. The diagnosis of acute pancreatitis depends on the serum amylase. A raised serum amylase can be seen in other abdominal emergencies (eg perforated duodenal ulcer), but if the amylase is more than five times greater than normal, acute pancreatitis is the most likely diagnosis.

3. B – Adenocarcinoma

The presence of malignant glandular cells on fine-needle aspiration is diagnostic of an adenocarcinoma. Adenocarcinoma is the most common pancreatic neoplasm and occurs most frequently in the elderly. Tumours in the head of the pancreas present with jaundice due to obstruction of the common bile duct. At first the jaundice is painless but as the disease progresses most patients experience some pain. Weight loss and anorexia also occur.

4. D – Chronic pancreatitis

Chronic pancreatitis is characterised by upper abdominal pain that develops gradually after heavy meals or bouts of heavy drinking. As in acute pancreatitis, the pain often radiates to the back and is relieved by leaning forwards. In this case, the abdominal calcification indicates chronic calcifying pancreatitis. This is the most common form in developed countries and is usually related to excess alcohol consumption. With repeated attacks of chronic pancreatitis, the pancreatic parenchyma is progressively destroyed, leading to pancreatic insufficiency and steatorrhoea. Diabetes mellitus eventually ensues due to destruction of the islets. The calcification seen on the radiograph is due to intraductal calculi.

5. H – Insulinoma

Insulinomas are pancreatic islet cell tumours that secrete insulin. The classic presenting feature is hypoglycaemia associated with fasting or exercise, although symptoms can occur at any time. Patients usually complain of episodic palpitations, dizziness, fainting, diplopia and confusion, but these are rather non-specific symptoms, so that misdiagnosis or delay in diagnosis is not uncommon. The diagnosis is made by demonstrating hypoglycaemia in association with inappropriate or excessive insulin secretion. Insulinomas are the most common type of islet cell tumour. They are usually solitary but can be very small and difficult to locate. Most tumours are cytologically benign.

ANSWERS TO CHAPTER – GENITOURINARY

1. ANATOMY OF THE GENITOURINARY SYSTEM

1. **H – Trigone of the bladder**
   The trigone is a triangular area of the bladder situated posteriorly. The base of the triangle lies between the two ureteric orifices and the apex passes down to the internal urethral opening. The mucosa over the area is smooth, contrasting with the folds elsewhere in the bladder. The trigone lies in front of the rectum, separated by the vagina in the female and by the vas deferens and seminal vesicles in the male.

2. **A – Body of the uterus**
   The fused Müllerian ducts form the uterus and upper vagina. The superolateral angles of the uterus give rise to the fallopian tubes on each side, which are overhung by pelvic folds of peritoneum. These folds and their contents form the broad ligaments and they, with the body of the uterus, form a partition across the pelvis, between the bladder anteriorly and the rectum posteriorly.

3. **D – Ovary**
   The ovarian fossa on the lateral wall of the pelvis lies below the external iliac vessels, bounded posteriorly by the ureter and internal iliac artery, and anteriorly by the obliterated umbilical artery. It is covered with peritoneum and overlies the obturator vessels and nerve. Medially, the ovary is surrounded by the infundibulum and fimbriae of the fallopian tube.

4. **F – Prostatic urethra**
   In the male the prostatic urethra is the widest part of the urethra. The ejaculatory ducts, formed by the union of the vas deferens and the openings of the seminal vesicles on each side, open onto an oval elevation (the verumontanum) on the posterior wall of the urethra. The median lobe of the prostate lies superior to the ejaculatory ducts. The two lateral lobes lie below and lateral to the median lobe; they are continuous anteriorly. The posterior union is palpable rectally as a posterior midline sulcus.

5. **C – Membranous urethra**
   The membranous urethra is the shortest and narrowest part of the male urethra. It is surrounded by the sphincter urethrae that fills most of the deep perineal pouch. The internal pudendal vessels and nerves and their branches lie within the pouch, and leave by piercing the underlying perineal membrane.

2. URINARY TRACT AND RELATED ANATOMY

1. **G – Right abdominal ureter**
   The abdominal ureter extends from the renal pelvis at the level of L2 (the left side usually being higher than the right) to the pelvic brim. The relations are the same in the male and female, but differ on the two sides. Both ureters lie on the psoas muscle and

cross the genitofemoral nerve. They are crossed by the gonadal vessels, on the right side by the root of the small gut mesentery and ileocolic artery, and on the left by the left colic artery and the sigmoid mesentery.

2. **A – Female pelvic ureter**
The pelvic ureters have the same relationships bilaterally, but differ in the male and female. Each ureter crosses the iliac vessels, in line with the sacroiliac joint, and descends to the ischial spine, where it turns forwards over the levator ani muscle to reach the bladder. In the male it is crossed by the vas deferens and in the female by the broad ligament. In the base of the broad ligament the ureter lies adjacent to the lateral fornix of the vagina.

3. **J – Right adrenal gland**
The adrenal glands lie on their respective crura of the diaphragm. The right is pyramidal in shape, capping the upper pole of the right kidney, and is tucked partly behind the inferior vena cava. The left is crescentic in shape, overlying the upper medial part of the kidney and renal pelvis. It is crossed by the splenic vessels and the tail of the pancreas.

4. **I – Right renal pelvis**
The second part of the duodenum crosses the right renal pelvis, the renal vessels passing to the hilum of the kidney lying between.

5. **D – Left renal pelvis**
The kidneys lie on the diaphragm, which separates them from the costodiaphragmatic recess and the lower two ribs. The psoas, quadratus lumborum and transverse abdominus muscles, and the subcostal, iliohypogastric and ilioinguinal nerves pass between. The anterior relations include the hepatic and splenic flexures of the colon.

3. HAEMATURIA I

1. **H – Prostate cancer**
This patient has prostatic cancer, as evidenced by the symptoms of bladder outflow obstruction and the high prostate-specific antigen (PSA) level (normal range is <6 nmol/l). The back pain could be due to metastatic disease. The bleeding is caused by erosion of a local vessel by tumour. Bleeding from the prostate and urethra (ie the distal urinary tract) is characteristically heaviest at the start of the urinary stream.

2. **B – Bladder cancer**
This patient has bladder carcinoma, as evidenced by the history. Bladder carcinoma must be considered to be the diagnosis in all cases of frank painless haematuria in older patients until proved otherwise. The occupational history might indicate exposure to aniline dyes, which are proved carcinogens in the context of bladder cancer. In addition, smoking leads to an increased risk of this disease. The diagnosis can be confirmed readily by urgent cystoscopy.

3. **G – Polycystic kidney disease**
This patient has polycystic kidney disease, this being strongly suggested by the finding of bilateral flank masses in association with haematuria. Other symptoms can include lumbar and abdominal pain, and the diagnosis is made by ultrasound scan or IVU.

Polycystic kidney disease is a common cause of chronic renal failure and this patient has a moderate degree of renal impairment. The disorder is inherited as an autosomal dominant trait and associations include polycystic disease of the liver and subarachnoid haemorrhage (from berry aneurysms).

4. I – Renal-cell carcinoma

This patient has a renal-cell carcinoma, as evidenced by the classic triad of haematuria, loin pain and abdominal mass. These tumours have a renal tubular cell origin and are adenocarcinomas. Other presentations include pyrexia of unknown origin (PUO) and night sweats, polycythaemia (2% of tumours secrete erythropoietin), anaemia and hypercalcaemia. The diagnosis is made by IVU, and staging is by computed tomography (CT). The mainstay of treatment is nephrectomy.

5. J – Ureteric calculus

This patient has a ureteric calculus that has led to ureteric colic, as evidenced by the acute onset of characteristic pain. The diagnosis is made by IVU. Emergency intervention (drainage) is only required in the presence of unilateral obstruction, if there is infection or deteriorating renal function, or the absence for any reason of a contralateral kidney.

4. HAEMATURIA II

1. D – Polycystic kidneys

This patient has adult polycystic kidney disease (APCKD). This is a relatively common autosomal dominant disorder and leads to end-stage renal failure in the third to fourth decades. The patient can present with haematuria secondary to an increased risk of urinary tract infections, renal stones, carcinoma or spontaneous bleeds into cysts.

2. E – Pyelonephritis

This patient has renal stones, which increases her risk of developing urinary tract infections and pyelonephritis. Without further investigations such as blood and urine cultures it is impossible to know what the causative agent is, and patients should be started on empirical antibiotics such as gentamicin and cephalosporins.

3. H – Renal tuberculosis

This patient has developed renal tuberculosis, as evidenced by the positive early-morning urine (EMU) sample. Such patients require a chest radiograph (to exclude metastases and confirm pulmonary tuberculosis), urine cytology, a midstream urine (MSU), three EMUs, and an ultrasound scan of the renal tract. Renal-cell carcinoma can present in a similar manner and is included in the differential diagnosis of a pyrexia of unknown origin (PUO).

4. F – Renal calculi

This patient has a renal stone in the left ureter that is causing obstruction. The MSU shows an aseptic pyuria, which is commonly caused by stones. Calculi can occur along the length of the renal tract but commonly occur within the renal pelvicalyceal system and bladder. They present with symptoms of obstruction, haematuria and infection. Predisposing factors to stone formation include abnormal anatomy (congenital abnormalities), abnormal and excess urinary tract excretion of stone-forming substances (eg oxalate, calcium, urate, cysteine) and chronic urinary tract infection. The majority of stone formation is idiopathic.

5. **B – *Escherichia coli* infection**
This elderly patient has developed an *Escherichia coli* urinary tract infection, as confirmed by the MSU result. Elderly patients can be apyrexial on admission and often have a relatively normal WCC. Clinical suspicion of sepsis should encourage the physician to treat empirically with antibiotics. Severe sepsis in the elderly carries significant risks and should be treated appropriately.

NB: Frank haematuria is pathological and requires investigation. The commonest cause is a urinary tract infection but after the age of 40 carcinoma and other causes should be excluded.

5. HYPOALBUMINAEMIA

1. **I – Septicaemia**
Severe illness, particularly sepsis, is a common cause of hypoalbuminaemia and this will not usually resolve until the underlying illness has been treated. A patient's admission serum albumin is a good guide to their general health, a subnormal albumin on admission being a poor prognostic indicator.

2. **C – Cirrhosis**
This patient has developed primary biliary cirrhosis (PBC) with secondary ascites. Her hypoalbuminaemia and raised international normalised ratio (INR) have occurred because her liver disease has led to an inability to synthesise vital proteins such as albumin, clotting factors and transport proteins.

3. **D – Malabsorption**
This patient has developed coeliac disease, with a macrocytic anaemia secondary to folate deficiency, and general malabsorption causing hypoalbuminaemia and steatorrhoea, which many people describe simply as 'diarrhoea'.

4. **H – Protein-losing enteropathy**
This man has developed a protein losing enteropathy secondary to Whipple's disease. Many serious, chronic conditions of the gastrointestinal tract can cause a protein-losing enteropathy. Whipple's disease characteristically presents with gastrointestinal disturbance, weight loss, arthralgia and anaemia and even finger clubbing, lymphadenopathy and peripheral oedema. It is a rare cause of gastrointestinal bleeding, endocarditis, pericarditis, pleurisy and papilloedema. The Gram-positive bacillus has now been identified and is grandly called *Tropheryma whippeli*.

5. **E – Malnutrition**
This patient has probable malnutrition secondary to anorexia nervosa. Her body mass index (BMI) is extremely low and she will require nutritional as well as psychiatric support.

NB: Hypoalbuminaemia is a reflection of the body's inability to absorb or synthesise protein or, as in nephrotic syndrome or protein-losing enteropathy, excess protein loss.

In normal pregnancy the total serum protein falls, principally due to a fall in serum albumin, although serum globulin levels rise. The mechanism of hypoalbuminaemia is still unclear.

6. GLOMERULONEPHRITIS

1. **A – Anti-glomerular basement membrane disease**
   This patient has anti-glomerular basement membrane disease, previously called 'Goodpasture's disease' or 'Goodpasture's syndrome' (see *EMQs Volume 1*, Chapter 5 – Respiratory, Theme 5: Haemoptysis). The glomerulonephritis is associated with an anti-glomerular basement membrane antibody (anti-GBM) that causes a nephrotic syndrome. The glomerular basement membrane shares a common antigenic component with the alveolar basement membrane, so the condition is associated with pulmonary haemorrhage (causing the pulmonary shadows on chest radiography). Goodpasture first described the condition in 1919 after the influenza pandemic that killed millions of people in 1918.

2. **G – Infective endocarditis**
   This patient has developed infective endocarditis, which can be associated with a rapidly progressive glomerulonephritis. The painful nodules in the pulps of the fingers are Osler's nodes. 'Rapidly progressive' describes the onset of end-stage renal failure (ESRF), which can occur within weeks or months of onset. Causes include malignancy, infection, the systemic vasculitides and anti-glomerular basement membrane disease.

3. **D – Henoch–Schönlein purpura**
   Henoch–Schönlein purpura is the association of palpable purpura, principally on the lower limbs and buttocks, a flitting arthritis, gut disturbances, including colicky abdominal pain and melaena, and glomerulonephritis. It can occur in children and in adults and is associated with ESRF in approximately 20–25% of cases, although the prognosis is better in children.

4. **F – Hodgkin's lymphoma**
   This patient has developed a glomerulonephritis secondary to lymphoma. The commonest associated type is minimal-change disease, but mesangiocapillary and membranous nephropathies have also been described. Lymphoma can also be associated with direct infiltration of the kidneys, rarely causing obstruction and cryoglobulinaemia. Therapy can cause a 'tumour lysis syndrome' due to the massive tumour cell destruction, which causes a severe uric acid nephropathy.

5. **B – Bronchial carcinoma**
   This man has bronchial carcinoma, which is mainly associated with membranous nephropathy.

7. CHRONIC INTERSTITIAL NEPHRITIS

1. G – NSAIDs

This patient has developed both upper gastrointestinal and renal tract side-effects of chronic non-steroidal anti-inflammatory drug (NSAID) use. NSAIDs have several toxic affects on the kidneys and can cause chronic interstitial nephritis and might also predispose patients to uro-epithelial tumours. Stopping the NSAIDs can lead to some recovery of the renal function.

2. C – Chronic pyelonephritis

This patient has developed chronic pyelonephritis or reflux nephropathy secondary to recurrent urinary tract infections. Patients of any age who present with recurrent urinary tract infections should be investigated with ultrasound and, if necessary, an IVU. Children need to have vesico-ureteric reflux excluded and older adults, tumours and calculi.

3. I – Sickle-cell disease

This gentleman has sickle-cell disease and has presented with an acute crisis secondary to a respiratory tract infection. Recurrent episodes typically cause renal ischaemic damage and tubular dysfunction and can lead to chronic renal failure (CRF). Renal failure is a major cause of morbidity in patients with sickle-cell disease who are aged over 40.

4. D – Diabetes mellitus

This man has developed diabetic nephropathy. He was probably diagnosed with impaired glucose tolerance or frank diabetes when he was diagnosed with ischaemic heart disease (IHD) but has not complied with treatment. His haemoglobin A_{1c} (Hb A_{1c}) reflects very poor control. Nephropathy in patients with IHD and diabetes mellitus can be retarded by the addition of an ACE inhibitor, which can slow progression towards ESRF and dialysis.

5. A – Alport's syndrome

This young boy has a rare, X-linked disorder known as 'Alport's syndrome'. This is the association of hereditary tubulointerstitial nephritis (causing ESRF), deafness and ocular abnormalities. It accounts for approximately 5% of childhood ESRF.

8. NEPHROTIC SYNDROME

1. H – Penicillamine

Penicillamine, like gold, is a disease-modifying agent of rheumatoid disease (DMARD), meaning that it has been shown to have a positive influence on both morbidity and prognosis. It is also used in primary biliary cirrhosis, Wilson's disease and heavy-metal poisoning. It is associated with numerous side-effects, including proteinuria, which is usually mild but can become severe enough to cause a nephrotic syndrome. The proteinuria is usually responsive to withdrawal of the penicillamine and to steroid therapy. Other causes of nephrotic syndrome in rheumatoid disease include amyloidosis and other therapies such as gold.

2. **E – IgA nephropathy**

    IgA nephropathy is the commonest cause of glomerulonephritis worldwide. It is principally found in young men in their second to third decade. The patients often have recurrent episodes of pharyngitis, associated with frank haematuria approximately 24–48 hours after their initial symptoms. Such episodes can be accompanied by myalgia, pyrexia, malaise and loin pains, mimicking a viral illness. The onset of the haematuria in relation to the pharyngitis differentiates it from post-streptococcal glomerulonephritis, which occurs 10–14 days after the onset of upper respiratory tract symptoms. There is at present no effective therapy and 1–3% of affected children and 25–40% of adults can progress to ESRF. In adults this can be many years after their initial presentation.

3. **J – Wegener's granulomatosis**

    This patient has the classica triad of upper and lower respiratory tract symptoms associated with renal impairment that is seen in Wegener's granulomatosis. The diagnosis is confirmed by the presence of the anti-proteinase 3 antibody and cytoplasmic antineutrophil cytoplasmic antibody (c-ANCA), which is present in 70–80% of untreated patients at presentation. The disease is characterised pathologically by a necrotising granulomatous vasculitis associated with a small-vessel renal vasculitis. The glomerulonephritis has an unpredictable onset and is often rapidly progressive.

4. **F – Malaria**

    This nephrotic syndrome is associated with falciparum malaria infection. The inclusion bodies are the intracellular trophozoites of the parasite. The nephrotic syndrome usually occurs in severe infection associated with haemolysis.

5. **G – Minimal-change nephropathy**

    Minimal-change nephropathy is a relatively common cause of nephrotic syndrome. It is so-called because light microscopy reveals no abnormalities and only electron microscopy can reveal the non-specific effacement of the epithelial podocytes. Patients' urinalyses characteristically shows a 'highly selective proteinuria'. It can be idiopathic or due to NSAIDs, Hodgkin's lymphoma or, more rarely, other carcinomas and anaphylaxis.

    NB: The nephrotic syndrome has many causes and is characterised by proteinuria of more than 3 g/24 hours, hypoalbuminaemia (<30 g/l) and peripheral oedema (although heavy proteinuria without peripheral oedema is now considered within this definition). Both micro- and macroscopic haematuria can occur but are not invariable. The oedema can include the upper extremeties and the face.

    Investigations in a patient suspected of having nephrotic syndrome should include a FBC, U&Es, albumin, ESR and vasculitis screen, chest radiography, a 24-hour urine collection to define proteinuria and creatinine clearance, renal ultrasound, and BP monitoring (and control). Common causes are:

    - Children: minimal change disease
    - Young adults: females – systemic lupus erythematossus (SLE); proliferative glomerulonephritis
    - Adults: diabetes mellitus, amyloidosis, membranous glomerulonephritis.

9. CALCIFICATION OF THE RENAL TRACT

1. **C – Hydatid cyst**
   This gentleman has previous hydatid disease, which is more common in sheep farmers and cattle farmers. The infection occurs when the larval stage of a canine tapeworm gets into the human food chain. This usually occurs through a dog excreting the tapeworm eggs and these being ingested by cattle and sheep, whose meat is then eaten by man. The eggs are absorbed into the circulation and are deposited into various viscera where they can develop into cysts: 70% occur in the liver, 20% in the lungs and 10% in various other sites, including the renal tract. Old cysts can involute and calcify.

2. **H – Schistosomiasis**
   This patient has developed schistosomiasis, a tropical fluke infection. Three species affect man, the main one infecting the renal tract being *Schistosoma haematobium*. Infection occurs through direct skin contact of the eggs in infected freshwater areas (eg lakes and rivers). The freshwater snail acts as an intermediary host. Renal tract effects include obstructive uropathy, nephrotic syndrome, calculi, pyelonephritis and squamous-cell carcinoma.

3. **J – Tuberculosis**
   This patient has evidence of old tuberculosis infection, which is probably not the cause of his pain. He has no evidence of acute infection.

4. **D – Hyperparathyroidism**
   This woman has hypercalcaemia due to hyperparathyroidism. Hypercalcaemia classically presents with 'moans, groans, bones and stones', ie depression, abdominal and other pains, bony swelling (late) and renal stones. Other common features include constipation, nausea and vomiting, dyspepsia, polyuria and polydipsia.

5. **I – Staghorn calculus**
   Recurrent *Proteus* renal tract infection predisposes patients to large 'staghorn' calculi. *Proteus* is a common cause of urinary tract infections but recurrent growth should alert the clinician to possible calculi and should prompt a renal tract ultrasound scan.

10. RENAL MASSES

1. **D – Polycystic kidney disease**
   This patient has adult polycystic kidney disease (APCKD). She has polycythaemia secondary to increased erythropoietin production and renal hypertension. Her other symptoms are principally related to her uraemia. The chromosomal abnormalities associated with this condition have been localised to several gene loci, including *PKD1* (short arm of chromosome 16) and *PKD2* (long arm of chromosome 4).

2. **F – Renal amyloidosis**
   This gentleman has renal amyloidosis associated with his chronic rheumatoid arthritis. Chronic conditions such as sepsis (eg tuberculosis), inflammatory conditions (eg the arthritides), and malignancy are associated with amyloid of the AA variant. The diagnosis can be confirmed by rectal biopsy or, in doubtful cases, renal biopsy.

3. **G – Renal-cell carcinoma**
   This patient has a nephroblastoma or Wilms' tumour (although first described by Rance in 1814!). It is a relatively common malignancy in the under-5s and accounts for 10% of all childhood malignancies. One in ten are bilateral and they classically present as a 'a large lump in a small (wasted) child'. Pain and haematuria are late manifestations. Several other congenital abnormalities are associated, including hemi-hypertrophy, exophthalmos and macroglossia. The prognosis has improved to 80–90% survival at 5 years due to the introduction of chemotherapy. Treatment includes nephrectomy, chemotherapy and, in metastatic disease, radiotherapy.

4. **A – Hydronephrosis**
   This patient has bilateral hydronephrosis secondary to bladder outflow tract obstruction. The symptoms and PSA suggest the likeliest cause is prostatic carcinoma.

5. **H – Renal cyst**
   This patient has a large renal cyst in the right kidney. Cysts are common, rarely cause symptoms and, as in this case, are often incidental findings on renal ultrasound scans. Rarely, they can be large enough to allow the kidney to be palpable. Patients can have several cysts in each kidney but this is not the same as polycystic kidney disease.

11. POLYCYSTIC KIDNEY DISEASE

1. **H – Subarachnoid haemorrhage**
   This patient has presented with a subarachnoid haemorrhage associated with rupture of a berry aneurysm. The hypertension and bradycardia are known as 'Cushing's reflex' and are associated with raised intracranial pressure. This patient needs to be intubated and ventilated, requires a confirmatory CT head scan, and should have intravenous nimodipine. Her prognosis is poor but you should discuss her management with a neurosurgical centre.

2. **C – Hypertension**
   This patient has hypertension associated with retinopathy. Hypertension is a common complication of all renal disease and must be tightly controlled to retard further deterioration in renal function. This patient requires review by a renal unit and her family should be screened for APCKD.

3. **D – Polycythaemia**
   Polycythaemia arises in APCKD as a result of increased renal production of erythropoietin. Treatment with regular venesection is required with the aim of keeping the haematocrit below 0.50.

4. **G – Renal-cell carcinoma**
   Adenocarcinoma is a relatively rare complication of APCKD. Haematuria and loin pain are more commonly caused by recurrent urinary tract infections and renal stones but these are excluded in this case by the urinalysis and MSU results.

5. **E – Recurrent urinary tract infection**
   This patient has developed pyelonephritis secondary to an *Eschrichia coli* urinary tract infection. Loin pain in patients with APCKD can be due to renal calculi, carcinoma,

bleeding into cysts or pyelonephritis, and the enlarging kidneys can also cause a non-specific dull ache.

12. TUMOURS OF THE URINARY TRACT

1. **F – Renal-cell carcinoma**
The triad of loin pain, haematuria and abdominal mass are the classic presenting features of a renal-cell carcinoma. Unfortunately they tend to be late manifestations and this accounts for the relatively poor prognosis. The fact that this lesion is poorly circumscribed and infiltrative signifies a malignant tumour. A diagnosis of renal-cell carcinoma is favoured by the location of the tumour, the macroscopic renal vein involvement and the clear-cell pattern on histology. The term 'adenocarcinoma' is sometimes used for renal parenchymal tumours, but this is a misnomer because the tumour does not produce mucin and is derived from tubular epithelium, not glandular epithelium.

2. **J – Transitional-cell carcinoma**
Transitional-cell carcinomas arise from the urothelium and can therefore be found in the bladder, ureters, renal pelvis and proximal urethra. They are strongly associated with exposure to certain carcinogens, particularly aniline dyes used in textiles and printing and reagents in the rubber, cable and plastic industries. Painless haematuria is the commonest presenting feature. Transitional-cell carcinomas are often multifocal and commonly have an exophytic, papillary growth pattern. Consequently, cells are frequently shed from the tumour surface into the urine, where they can be detected on cytological examination as atypical or frankly malignant cells.

3. **D – Nephroblastoma**
Nephroblastoma, or Wilms' tumour, is the commonest intra-abdominal tumour in children and has a peak incidence between 1 year and 4 years of age. The most frequent presentation is with an abdominal mass, though haematuria and hypertension are also common. The tumour is derived from mesonephric mesoderm and histologically has both epithelial and mesenchymal tissues, with a rather primitive or embryonic appearance. The tumour is rapidly growing and behaves aggressively.

4. **I – Squamous-cell carcinoma**
Squamous-cell carcinomas of the bladder arise in metaplastic squamous epithelium. This change occurs as a result of chronic irritation and inflammation of the bladder mucosa, usually due to calculi or infection with *Schistosoma haematobium*. In parts of Africa and the Middle East schistosomiasis is endemic and consequently squamous-cell carcinoma of the bladder is common. Like squamous-cell carcinomas elsewhere, those arising in the bladder show a range of differentiation; keratin is found in the better-differentiated lesions. Squamous cell carcinomas of the bladder are usually solid and invasive rather than papillary and so have a worse prognosis than transitional-cell carcinomas.

5. **B – Angiomyolipoma**
Angiomyolipoma is an intrarenal mass that, as its name implies, is composed of a mixture of blood vessels, muscle and mature fat. It is probably a hamartoma, rather than a true neoplasm. Like other benign renal tumours, it is usually asymptomatic and found incidentally. Angiomyolipoma is present in 25–50% of patients with tuberose

sclerosis, an inherited disorder with malformations of the central nervous system, eye, skin and other viscera.

13. RENAL FAILURE

1. **E – Haemorrhage**
    This patient has had an upper gastrointestinal bleed secondary to his alcoholic liver disease. The most common causes include peptic ulcer disease, oesophageal and gastric varices, and alcoholic gastritis. The patient has pre-renal failure as evidenced by the markedly raised urea in comparison with the mildly elevated creatinine. An element of this raised urea will be due to the absorption of the protein from blood within the gut lumen. Other markers of his chronic alcoholic liver disease include macrocytosis, thrombocytopenia and hyponatraemia (due to secondary hyperaldosteronism).

2. **B – Carcinoma of the prostate**
    This man has developed obstructive renal impairment secondary to prostatic carcinoma. The passage of a urinary catheter either urethrally or suprapubically will relieve the obstruction but he will require urological transurethral resection. His back pain is a sinister symptom and requires investigation with plain radiographs and an isotope bone scan. Therapeutic interventions include surgery, anti-androgens and radiotherapy.

3. **I – Renal artery stenosis**
    This patient has developed acute renal failure secondary to her ACE inhibitor. Peripheral vascular disease is commonly associated with significant atherosclerotic renal artery stenosis and is a contraindication for the initiation of ACE inhibitors. This woman has symptoms and signs of uraemia. Other common symptoms include nausea and vomiting, hiccups, pericarditis, seizures and decreasing level of consciousness.

4. **J – Rhabdomyolysis**
    This elderly patient has developed a 'crush injury' from lying on the floor for 72 hours. Whatever the cause of her fall (which will need investigation) she has now developed rhabdomyolysis-induced renal failure. The diagnosis is confirmed by myoglobinuria. Treatment includes central venous access, strict fluid balance, maintenance of adequate venous pressures (>10 cm of water), urinary catheterisation and expert renal management. Patients are often treated with empirical broad-spectrum antibiotics.

5. **F – Henoch–Schönlein purpura**
    This man has developed Henoch–Schönlein purpura (HSP) with its associated membranous nephropathy. HSP is characterised by purpura of the extensor surfaces of the lower and upper limbs and buttocks, with sparing of the face and trunk. The purpura can become palpable and is associated with an arthritis, gastrointestinal symptoms and a glomerulonephritis. The diagnosis is usually made by the association of these manifestations and can be confirmed by skin or renal biopsy, which characteristically shows the presence of IgA and C3 by immunofluorescence. Approximately 50% of patients have raised serum IgA levels.

14. CRYOGLOBULINAEMIA AND RENAL FAILURE

1. **I – Sjögren's syndrome**
This patient has Sjögren's syndrome with an associated mixed cryoglobulinaemia. She has the classic triad of arthralgia, skin and renal involvement. The treatment of such a patient includes steroids and cytotoxins; plasmapheresis is sometimes required.

2. **D – Leptospirosis**
This man has developed leptospirosis, a spirochaetal infection. The infection has two phases, an acute phase and, several days later, an immune phase. The vast majority of patients recover with few complications but some develop a severe illness associated with a haemolytic anaemia, jaundice, renal and even cardiac failure. Antibiotic treatment includes penicillin, erythromycin or tetracycline.

3. **C – Infective endocarditis**
This patient has developed bacterial endocarditis with a secondary cryoglobulinaemia. Unlike the examples in scenarios 1 and 2, this is a type II cryoglobulinaemia, principally associated with infective processes (eg cytomegalovirus [CMV], Epstein–Barr virus [EBV], hepatitis B virus [HBV] and hepatitis C virus [HCV] infections).

4. **A – Epstein–Barr virus**
This young man has developed glandular fever caused by EBV. This can be associated with a type II cryoglobulinaemia, although this complications is rare.

5. **J – Waldenström's macroglobulinaemia**
This gentleman has Waldenström's macroglobulinaemia, as evidenced by his ESR, the presence of lymphoplasmacytoid cells in the bone marrow and the IgM paraproteinaemia. The absence of hypercalcaemia or lytic lesions in the bones makes multiple myeloma unlikely.

15. NEPHROTOXIC DRUGS

1. **A – Amphotericin B**
Amphotericin B is used in severe systemic fungal infections. These are more common in immunosuppressed patients, as in this case. When given intravenously it commonly causes toxicity. It can cause hypokalaemia, hypomagnesaemia and renal failure. Less toxic, more lipid-soluble formulations are now available that are less nephrotoxic.

2. **D – Gentamicin**
Gentamicin is both nephrotoxic and ototoxic as it is preferentially absorbed into the vestibular and renal tissues. It has a narrow therapeutic window and must therefore be carefully monitored. Toxicity is common when subtherapeutic doses are maintained over several days or with pre-existing dehydration or renal impairment. It is recommended that in healthy adults a dose of 3–5 mg/kg is used as an initial dose with once-daily or twice-daily dosing used thereafter. With pre-existing renal impairment or in elderly patients, the initial dose should be 1–2 mg/kg.

3. **E – Gold**
    Gold is one of the DMARDs and is used in an intramuscular injection or in tablet form. It has numerous side-effects, including nephrotic syndrome, pulmonary fibrosis, hepatotoxicity, photosensitivity and agranulocytosis.

4. **I – Perindopril**
    ACE inhibitors are commonly associated with a mild derangement of the U&Es in the elderly but usually this does not have any clinical significance. In patients with generalised atherosclerotic disease, particularly peripheral vascular disease, or with bilateral renal artery stenosis, the ACE inhibitors can cause fulminant acute renal failure.

5. **B – Co-trimoxazole**
    This patient has developed *Pneumocystis carinii* pneumonia (PCP) and has been started on co-trimoxazole. This contains sulfamethoxazole and trimethoprim. The drug has numerous side-effects, including pancytopenia, hepatotoxicity, seizures and ataxia. It is nephrotoxic and can cause a spectrum of problems from mild electrolyte disturbance to interstitial nephritis.

16. RENAL MANIFESTATIONS OF SYSTEMIC DISEASE

1. **H – Sickle-cell disease**
    Sickle cell disease can be associated with frank haematuria in an acute sickling crisis due to infection or as a direct result of ischaemic insults within the renal pelvicalyceal system. Other renal manifestations in sickle-cell disease include nocturnal enuresis in childhood (the cause being unclear) and acute membranoproliferative glomerulonephritis leading to a nephrotic syndrome. Chronic renal failure is a significant contributor to morbidity and mortality in the over-40s.

2. **G – Sarcoidosis**
    This patient has sarcoidosis. Sarcoid can affect the kidney in several ways, including nephrocalcinosis, renal stones, acute and chronic interstitial nephritis, amyloidosis, membranous glomerulonephropathy and hypertension. Direct infiltrations with granuloma are associated with extrarenal disease and often present insidiously with moderate to severe renal impairment, as in this case.

3. **I – Systemic lupus erythematosus**
    This patient has developed 'lupus nephritis', which occurs in approximately 50% of patients with adult SLE. It occurs more commonly in women and in young adults aged 15–25 years. The World Health Organisation (WHO) classification of lupus nephritis defines the underlying histological changes on light microscopy and in this way defines treatment and prognosis. Treatment includes steroids for all patients and, in the more 'malignant' types (types III and IV), immunosuppression with azathioprine, cyclophosphamide or methotrexate. In most cases the condition 'burns out' within 5 years and few patients progress to ESRF.

Type	Glomerular change	Proportion of total no. of cases
I	Virtually normal histology	0–5%
II	Mesangial	15–20%
IIIA	Focal	20–30%
IIIB	Slightly more diffuse	
IV	Diffuse	45–60%
V	Membranous	10–15%

4. **A – Crohn's disease**
This patient has Crohn's disease, which can be associated with oxalate renal stones, particularly after small-bowel resection. This patient has presented with pyelonephritis secondary to his stones. Treatment should include intravenous fluids and antibiotics. Crohn's disease can also cause renal amyloidosis, subsequent nephrotic syndrome and renal failure.

5. **D – Hepatitis C**
Hepatitis B and hepatitis C can both cause glomerulonephritis and a nephrotic syndrome. HBV is a DNA virus and is identified by the presence of HBs antigen; HCV is an RNA virus. Both are blood-borne and can be contracted from blood products, sexual intercourse and intravenous drug use.

17. URINARY INCONTINENCE

1. **I – Spinal cord compression**
This patient has signs and symptoms consistent with spinal cord compression secondary to her metastatic carcinoma. This can present with relatively insidious symptoms, including sensory and motor loss in the limbs, constipation and incontinence. The incontinence is overflow incontinence secondary to a 'neurogenic'/atonic bladder. This patient needs neurosurgical decompression of the cord.

2. **G – Normal-pressure hydrocephalus**
This elderly man has the classic triad of normal-pressure hydrocephalus (ie confusion, incontinence and gait dyspraxia) leading to falls. The name of this condition is in fact a misnomer because it is thought that such patients have a varying cerebrospinal fluid (CSF) pressure through the day, with periods of high and normal pressures. A CT head scan might confirm dilated ventricles with relative sparing of the sulci. Neurosurgical insertion of a ventriculo-peritoneal shunt might improve the symptoms; patients with all three features of the triad seem to benefit the most from surgical intervention.

3. **C – Detrusor instability**
Detrusor instability is causing this patient's incontinence. This can be associated with prostatic hypertrophy but this is unlikely in this case as the patient has had a prostatic resection and his symptoms improve with an anticholinergic. Patients require a bladder

ultrasound before and after micturition to define the residual volume in their bladder. If the residual volume is less than 100 ml they can safely be given an anticholinergic. Symptoms for those with a residual volume of more than 100 ml would get worse with this treatment because anticholinergics cause retention and stasis.

4. **A – Benign prostatic hypertrophy**
    This patient probably has benign prostatic hypertrophy that is causing bladder outflow tract obstruction. Alpha-blockers such as terazosin relax the smooth muscle at the neck of the bladder, aiding voiding. Despite treatment, these symptoms can progress, and a transurethral resection of prostate (TURP) might be required.

5. **J – Urinary tract infection**
    This elderly woman has a urinary tract infection. This type of sepsis is a common cause of illness in the elderly and can present in numerous ways, including progressive incontinence.

18. URINARY TRACT OBSTRUCTION I

1. **E – Renal stones**
    This patient has recurrent *Proteus* infection that predisposes her to staghorn caluli. These are large irregular renal stones that are radio-opaque and can cause renal tract obstruction.

2. **D – Prostatic carcinoma**
    This gentleman has a history suggestive of metastatic carcinoma of the prostate. This can cause obstruction locally, leading to an obstructed bladder and proximal urinary tract or can cause a neurogenic bladder through cord compression secondary to metastases. The latter is excluded by his normal neurological assessment.

3. **F – Retroperitoneal fibrosis**
    Retroperitoneal fibrosis is a relatively rare cause of urinary tract obstruction. It is idiopathic in the majority of cases but can be associated with malignancy (as in this case), inflammatory processes such as Crohn's disease, appendicitis and diverticulitis, and abdominal aortic aneurysm. It is also associated with the use of methysergide.

4. **B – Myelomatous light chains**
    This gentleman has a grossly elevated ESR, hypercalcaemia and lytic bone lesions on his radiographs. These are all highly suggestive of multiple myeloma. Myeloma can cause renal failure for several reasons, including light-chain obstruction of the tubules, nephrocalcinosis, glomerulonephritis and pre-renal dehydration.

5. **C – Neurogenic bladder**
    A neurogenic bladder arises due to interruption of the complex neurological supply to the bladder. This can be in the central nervous system, associated with stroke, tumours, demyelination and cord compression, or peripherally, when associated with direct invasion or damage to the sacral plexus. In this patient, bony metastases have caused spinal cord compression.

19. URINARY TRACT OBSTRUCTION II

1. **B – Benign prostatic hypertrophy**
    This patient is most likely to have benign prostatic hypertrophy (BPH) as evidenced by the history and examination findings. While a raised PSA is usually indicative of carcinoma of the prostate, a small rise (as in this case) often also occurs with BPH.

2. **F – Neurogenic bladder**
    The cause of this patient's chronic retention of urine is autonomic neuropathy secondary to diabetes mellitus. The bladder becomes atonic after acute lesions of the spinal cord or cauda equina and remains atonic during the period of spinal shock, which in humans lasts for several weeks. It also becomes atonic with pure sensory lesions such as tabes dorsalis and in some of the sacral autonomic neuropathies such as those caused by diabetes. In contrast, the automatic bladder empties spontaneously with small degrees of filling, and is caused by lack of upper motor neurone inhibition. This therefore occurs in central nervous system lesions including spinal cord injury after spinal shock has resolved.

3. **D – Clot retention**
    This gentleman has clot retention, as evidenced by the history of bladder cancer with frank haematuria. Bladder cancer can itself cause direct bladder outflow obstruction if the tumour obstructs the urethral outflow, but clot retention is a more likely cause of acute retention in this case. Normal catheters often become rapidly blocked by clot, so a larger three-way irrigation catheter is usually required until the haematuria resolves.

4. **H – Prostatic oedema**
    The cause of this patient's acute retention of urine is prostatic oedema. An acute presentation with few previous symptoms is not uncommon after surgery in the pelvic region, which can be complicated by oedema of the prostate gland. It is more likely in patients with known prostatic enlargement, however. Patients at risk should be warned in the context of giving consent for the operation if there is a risk of the need for post-operative urethral catheterisation.

5. **I – Urethral stricture**
    This patient has an urethral stricture. After prostatic causes, this is probably the commonest cause of bladder outflow obstruction. Causes include rare congenital conditions, inflammation (usually secondary to infection), urethral carcinoma (rare in the UK), balanitis xerotica obliterans and trauma. While acute trauma to the membranous urethra as a result of pelvic fractures or other trauma is important, far more numerous are strictures which follow damage to the urethra by indwelling catheters, as in this case. Suprapubic catheterisation will be required for a patient in acute retention like this

20. SCROTAL SWELLINGS

1. **D – Idiopathic (primary) hydrocele**
    This patient has idiopathic hydrocele, as evidenced by the history and examination findings. A hydrocele is an abnormal quantity of serous fluid (hence transilluminable) within the tunica vaginalis (which is why the testis is impalpable). Primary, idiopathic hydroceles usually occur in men over the age of 40 and develop slowly, becoming

large and eventually tense. Hydroceles can also occur secondary to infection, trauma or malignancy. These usually appear more rapidly and will usually be associated with symptoms of the underlying disorder.

2. **H – Testicular torsion**
    This patient has torsion of the testis, as evidenced by the patient's age, classic history and examination findings. The commonest age for torsion is between 10 years and 15 years (it very rarely occurs over 21 years). It is, however, sometimes difficult to distinguish a torsion from acute epididymo-orchitis in sexually active young males. While the two can usually be clinically separated, surgical exploration is mandatory if there is any doubt over the diagnosis, in order to prevent loss of the testis.

3. **G – Testicular teratoma**
    This is a testicular teratoma, as evidenced by the age of the patient, history and exami-nation findings, as well as the tumour markers. Teratomas are germ-cell tumours which most commonly occur in 20–30-year-olds. In contrast, seminoma, the other common testicular malignancy, occurs in an older age group (30–40 years). Both present as a painless swelling or lump in the testis which is palpable as a hard irregular mass in patients where a secondary hydrocele is absent (see above). Alpha-fetoprotein (αFP) is produced by yolk-sac cellular elements and is raised in teratoma but not in seminoma. Beta-human chorionic gonadotrophin (β-hCG) is secreted by trophoblastic cells and can be present in either tumour type.

4. **B – Acute epididymo-orchitis**
    This is acute epididymo-orchitis, as evidenced by the history and examination findings. Epididymo-orchitis is inflammation, usually primarily of the epididymis, most commonly bacterial. In younger men, it is usually secondary to sexually transmitted diseases such as *Chlamydia* or gonorrhoea (torsion must be excluded – see above). It also commonly occurs in an older age group, when it is secondary to urinary tract infection with coliforms.

5. **A – Acute haematocele**
    This is an acute haematocele, as evidenced by the history of trauma and examination findings. A haematocele is a collection of blood within the tunica vaginalis. Acute haematocele is a common accompaniment of scrotal trauma, but a secondary haema-tocele can also occur with infection and tumours of the testis. In either case it can be distinguished from a hydrocele because it does not transilluminate. If left untreated, the resultant haematoma can form a hard, non-tender mass, which is clinically indistin-guishable from a testicular tumour.

21. MENORRHAGIA

1. **C – Fibroids**
    Fibroids are leiomyomas of the uterus, a benign tumour of the smooth muscle. They can present as an abdominal mass, painless menorrhagia, infertility problems and, more rarely, pain, due to torsion or 'red degeneration' during pregnancy. They are common and occur in 5% of women, the frequency increasing with age. They are classified anatomically as subserous, intramural, submucosal or cervical. Rarely, they can undergo malignant sarcomatous change.

2. **A – Adenomyosis**
Endometrial tissue can occur ectopically within and outside the uterus, a process known as 'endometriosis'. Uterine endometriosis, occurring within the myometrium, can be localised (adenomyoma), or more diffuse, causing a fibromyomatous reaction known as 'adenomyosis'. This diffuse reaction commonly causes painful menorrhagia and the patient requires a hysterectomy.

3. **G – Physiological**
'Physiological' menorrhagia is a diagnosis of exclusion. It is commonly experienced by women who have recently stopped taking the oral contraceptive pill, who are used to regular, relatively light periods. The diagnosis can only be made after local lesions and blood dyscrasias have been excluded.

4. **F – Pelvic inflammatory disease**
This patient has acute on chronic pelvic inflammatory disease caused by chlamydial infection. Acute episodes can be marked by abdominal pain, tenderness and fever and, on examination, a positive cervical excitation test and adnexal tenderness. An endo-cervical smear might identify the causative organisms but some patients require a laparoscopy to confirm the diagnosis. Patients should be treated with broad-spectrum antibiotics such as doxycycline, metronidazole or ciprofloxacin.

5. **J – von Willebrand's disease**
This girl has von Willebrand's disease, an autosomal dominant disorder, caused by a defective gene on chromosome 12. Patients have defective or deficient factor VIII:von Willebrand's factor (VIII:vWF), which in turn leads to defective platelet aggregation and factor VIII:c deficiency. Patients usually have a long history of prolonged bleeding after minor trauma, epistaxis or menorrhagia. In severe cases, patients can require factor VIII concentrate but most only need prophylaxis for surgical procedures.

22. INTERMENSTRUAL BLEEDING

1. **A – Cervical carcinoma**
Cervical carcinoma is a common cancer in women and despite mass screening using cervical smear tests, the incidence has not changed dramatically. It is a disease of middle age but can occur in women as young as 30. Histologically, it is principally a squamous carcinoma but can also be an adenocarcinoma and, very rarely, a sarcoma. Risk factors include multiple sexual partners, early age of coitus and human papillomavirus (HPV) serotypes 13, 18, 31 and 33. The prognosis depends on the stage of the disease, with 5-year survival rates of >90% for stage I disease (microinvasive), 55% for stage II disease (spread beyond the cervix), and <10% for stage IV disease (involving pelvic structures and distal metastases).

2. **G – Endometriosis**
Endometriosis has been described in multiple sites around the pelvis, abdomen and even within the thorax. The symptoms are related to the various sites, menstrual irregularity (peri-ovarian), dysmenorrhoea and deep dyspareunia (within the pouch of Douglas) and menorrhagia and infertility (within the myometrium). Laparoscopy is the definitive diagnostic method and can also be used to apply diathermy to local areas. Symptoms often improve with pregnancy and medical therapy is aimed at producing a

'pseudopregnancy' using continuous progestagens, the combined oral contraceptive pill or danazol, a steroid used to suppress gonadotrophin secretion. In severe cases hysterectomy with bilateral salpingo-oophorectomy might be required.

3. **F – Endometrial carcinoma**
Endometrial carcinoma is a relatively rare cause of intermenstrual bleeding because it is rare before the age of 40; the median age of onset is 60. As in this case it can occur perimenopausally and create a very difficult diagnostic picture. It must be excluded in all post-menopausal women presenting with vaginal bleeding. In pre-menopausal women it is a cause of intermenstrual bleeding. Risk factors include early menarche/late menopause, nulliparity, obesity and a previous history of cervical and ovarian carcinoma.

4. **B – Cervical ectropion**
This patient has a cervical ectropion (previously called an 'erosion'). This can arise spontaneously in adolescence or during pregnancy, in those on the oral contraceptive pill or due to a cervical tear. It is caused by the endocervical epithelium proliferating distally, extending over the ectocervical epithelium. It is often asymptomatic and only discovered on routine examination but can be a cause of bleeding, vaginal discharge or infection. Most patients require no intervention but cryotherapy is required in more florid cases.

5. **E – Ectopic pregnancy**
This patient has signs, symptoms and investigations suggestive of an ectopic pregnancy. This is an obstetric emergency and requires rapid diagnosis and treatment. The history in a sexually active woman of lower abdominal pain, amenorrhoea, and vaginal bleeding is highly suggestive of an ectopic pregnancy. Patients can require resuscitation with fluids and blood and emergency laparoscopy. Diagnosis is confirmed by a positive pregnancy test and an ultrasound scan of the uterus which excludes an intrauterine gestational sac, although this can be difficult in the very early stages when the gestational sac is not visible. Approximately 95% of cases occur in the fallopian tubes and laparoscopy should be aimed at removing the pregnancy and, if possible, preserving the tube.

23. SECONDARY AMENORRHOEA

1. **J – Prolactinoma**
This woman has a microadenoma of the pituitary gland, which is causing hyperprolactinaemia and secondary amenorrhoea. Microadenomas are less than 1 cm in diameter and cause a rise in serum prolactin to 2000 mU/l. Higher levels can occur with lactotroph macroadenomas and other large pituitary masses which cause interference with the hypothalamic-pituitary stalk, thus removing the inhibitory effects of hypothalamic dopamine. Microadenomas present with loss of libido, infertility and galactorrhoea, but not with local pressure effects, which are suggestive of larger pituitary masses.

2. **H – Polycystic ovary syndrome**
This patient has several of the features of polycystic ovary syndrome. She has hirsutism, obesity and amenorrhoea. The rise in serum luteinising hormone (LH) causes a rise in androstenedione, which is converted peripherally to testosterone. The diagnosis is confirmed by the biochemical changes and ultrasound scan of the ovaries, which

shows polycystic disease. Treatment includes weight loss, cyproterone (an androgen antagonist) or the combined oral contraceptive pill.

3. **B – Anorexia nervosa**
    Severe malnutrition and low BMI both lead to amenorrhoea. Her blood tests reveal a macrocytic anaemia, folate deficiency and hypoalbuminaemia, indicating chronic malnutrition.

4. **C – Congenital adrenal hyperplasia**
    Congenital adrenal hyperplasia comprises a group of disorders leading to abnormal adrenal steroid metabolism. The commonest form of the condition is due to 21α-hydroxylase deficiency. The net effect is that cortisol and aldosterone production is diverted, due to the enzyme deficiencies, into adrenal sex hormone synthesis. In the severe form, neonates present with ambiguous genitalia and adrenal insufficiency. In the more benign forms, female patients present in early adolescence with premature development of pubic hair and later with amenorrhoea and hirsutism. Biochemically, 21α-hydroxylase deficiency is characterised by an excess of serum and urinary 17α-hydroxyprogesterone.

5. **G – Panhypopituitarism**
    This patient has developed panhypopituitarism secondary to Sheehan`s syndrome. Sheehan`s syndrome is due to post-partum infarction of the pituitary and is usually associated with a massive post-partum haemorrhage or other cause of prolonged post-partum hypotension. Patients present with non-specific symptoms, such as malaise and lethargy, and specific symptoms associated with the hormonal deficiencies. Treatment includes hormone replacement therapy with gonadal steroids, cortisol and thyroxine.

24. PRURITUS VULVAE

1. **H – Vaginal warts**
    This patient has developed vulval warts, which are spread through sexual contact. They are caused by the human papillomavirus (HPV), which has been linked to the development of both vulval and cervical carcinoma. The warts can occur on the vulva, vagina and cervix, as well as the perineum and anus. Treatment should include the exclusion of other sexually transmitted diseases, contact tracing and local diathermy, cryotherapy or laser treatment.

2. **D – Gonorrhoea**
    This patient has developed gonorrhoea, another sexually transmitted disease. It is caused by *Neisseria gonorrhoeae*, a Gram-negative diplococcus. The infection should be treated with co-trimoxazole, ciprofloxacin or penicillin and probenecid. As with all sexually transmitted infections contact tracing should be arranged.

3. **J – Vulval dystrophy**
    Vulval dystrophy is the term given to a group of disorders that present with pruritus vulvae and vulval atrophy. They are differentiated by biopsy, which might show a hyperplastic, hypoplastic or mixed architecture. The three histological types can also include areas of atypia which can become malignant. Hypoplastic areas should be treated with topical oestrogens whereas hypertrophic areas require treatment with topical steroids.

4. **F – Trichomoniasis**
    Trichomoniasis is a sexually transmitted disease caused by the flagellate protozoan, *Trichomonas vaginalis*. In women it typically causes an offensive, frothy, greenish vaginal discharge with an associated cervicitis and pruritus and can even cause cystitis. In contrast, in affected men it is often asymptomatic. Treatment includes metronidazole and contact tracing.

5. **B, C – Candidiasis and diabetes mellitus**
    This patient has developed type 2 diabetes mellitus, as indicated by her raised glycosylated haemoglobin (Hb A_{1c}). Because of her diabetes she has subsequently developed vaginal candidiasis, which should be treated with clotrimazole cream and/or pessaries.

25. NEOPLASMS OF THE FEMALE GENITAL TRACT

1. **F – Mature cystic teratoma**
    Germ-cell tumours constitute 15–20% of all ovarian tumours and arise from oocytes. The most common germ-cell tumour is the mature cystic teratoma, also known as a 'dermoid cyst'. They are usually found in young women during the active reproductive years, though they can occur at any age. Typically, mature cystic teratomas are smooth-walled unilocular cysts that contain sebaceous material, hair and teeth. Histologically, they show a wide range of mature tissues, such as skin, bronchial epithelium, intestinal epithelium, cartilage and bone. These tumours are benign, though very rarely one of the component elements, usually squamous epithelium, can undergo malignant transformation.

2. **A – Adenocarcinoma**
    The endometrium is composed both of glands and stroma: in this patient it is the glandular element that has undergone malignant transformation and the tumour is therefore an adenocarcinoma. Clinical features associated with this tumour include obesity, diabetes mellitus, hypertension and nulliparity. There are two clinicopathological types of endometrial adenocarcinoma: one arises on a background of endometrial hyperplasia as a result of unopposed oestrogen activity; the other arises in atrophic postmenopausal endometrium. The prognosis of this tumour depends on the extent of myometrial invasion at the time of diagnosis.

3. **I – Squamous-cell carcinoma**
    The vulva is lined by keratinised, stratified squamous epithelium and the majority of malignant tumours arising in the vulva are therefore squamous-cell carcinomas. In this patient, the macroscopic appearance of the ulcer – with raised, rolled, everted edges – suggests malignancy, and squamous-cell carcinoma is confirmed by finding invasive tumour islands producing keratin. The enlarged inguinal lymph nodes imply metastatic nodal disease. Squamous-cell carcinoma of the vulva is a tumour of elderly women and usually presents late in its clinical course. Its histological appearance and behaviour are similar to those of squamous-cell carcinoma at other sites.

4. **E – Leiomyoma**
    The uterine leiomyoma is the most common benign tumour of the female genital tract. The term 'fibroid' is a misnomer because these lesions arise from myometrial smooth muscle. The peak incidence is in late reproductive life or around the time of the

menopause. Common presenting features include abdominal mass, irregular uterine bleeding and infertility. Typically, leiomyomas are multiple, round, well-circumscribed masses that range in diameter from 0.5 cm to 20 cm or more, often causing substantial distortion of the uterus. Histologically, they are composed of interlacing bundles of smooth-muscle fibres showing little or no mitotic activity.

5. **C – Dysgerminoma**

    Dysgerminoma is an undifferentiated germ-cell tumour that is the ovarian counterpart of testicular seminoma. It is proportionately less common than seminoma, though, like seminoma, it has a peak incidence in young adults and is usually unilateral and solid. Histologically, it is also very similar to seminoma, with large 'undifferentiated' germ cells with prominent nucleoli, admixed with numerous lymphocytes. It behaves as a malignant tumour and is radiosensitive.

ANSWERS TO CHAPTER – MUSCULOSKELETAL

1. CUTANEOUS INNERVATION OF THE UPPER LIMB

1. **B – Axillary nerve**
    The upper lateral cutaneous nerve of the arm supplying the skin over deltoid is a branch of the axillary nerve. The axillary nerve can be damaged in dislocation of the shoulder joint and fractures of the surgical neck of the humerus. Immediately post-injury, the sensory loss is easier to assess than paralysis of the deltoid muscle.

2. **C – Medial cutaneous nerve of the forearm**
    The medial cutaneous nerve of the forearm pierces the deep fascia in the mid upper arm with the basilic vein, and supplies the skin over the medial aspect of lower arm and forearm to the wrist.

3. **I – Radial nerve**
    The radial nerve passes under cover of the brachioradialis in the forearm and crosses the scaphoid fossa. It innervates the skin over the posterior aspect of the hand, and the lateral two and a half digits, as far as the nail bed.

4   **D – Median nerve**
    The median nerve supplies the lateral palm and skin over the anterior aspect, the tip and the nail bed of the lateral two and a half digits.

5. **J – Ulnar nerve**
    The ulnar nerve supplies the anterior and posterior aspects of the medial side of the hand, and the palmar one and a half, and dorsal three and a half fingers, through its palmar and dorsal branches.

The anterior and posterior interosseus nerves are deeply placed in the forearm and have no cutaneous innervation. The musculocutaneous nerve pierces the deep fascia on the lateral side of the biceps tendon to become the lateral cutaneous nerve of the forearm, supplying the lateral skin down to the wrist. The posterior cutaneous nerves of the arm and forearm supply the posterior aspect of the upper limb from the axilla to the wrist. They are branches of the radial nerve arising respectively in the axilla and over the radial groove of the humerus.

2. NERVE SUPPLY OF THE MUSCLES OF THE UPPER LIMB

1. **D – Lower subscapular nerve**
    The lower subscapular nerve also supplies the subscapularis muscle.

2. **I – Radial nerve**
   After piercing the lateral intermuscular septum, the radial nerve also supplies the extensor carpi radialis longus and brevis, before dividing into the posterior interosseus nerve and the radial cutaneous nerve. The latter passes distally deep to the brachioradialis muscle.

3. **H – Posterior interosseus nerve**
   The posterior interosseus nerve passes between the heads of the supinator muscle and supplies the deep extensor muscles of the forearm.

4. **J – Ulnar nerve**
   The ulnar nerve enters the forearm between the heads of flexor carpi ulnaris. It also supplies the medial half of flexor digitorum profundus, the hypothenar and interosseus muscles, the medial two lumbricals and the adductor pollicis muscle.

5. **F – Median nerve**
   The median nerve passes between the heads of the pronator teres and deep to the flexor digitorum sublimus in the forearm. It supplies these muscles, together with flexor carpi radialis, palmus longus, the thenar muscles except adductor pollicis, and the lateral two lumbricals.

   The anterior interosseus nerve is a branch of the median nerve and supplies flexor pollicis longus, half of flexor digitorum profundus and pronator quadratus. The axillary nerve supplies deltoid and teres minor muscles, and the lateral aspect of the upper arm over the deltoid muscle. The long thoracic nerve supplies serratus anterior and the musculocutaneous nerve supplies brachialis, biceps and corocobrachialis before becoming the lateral cutaneous nerve of the forearm. The medial cutaneous nerve of the forearm passes through the deep fascia with the basilic vein to supply the medial aspect of the lower arm and forearm to the wrist.

3. MUSCLE ATTACHMENTS OF THE FOREARM

1. **C – Brachioradialis**
   The distal attachment of the brachioradialis is to the lateral aspect of the lower end of the radius. The muscle flexes the elbow joint most effectively in mid-pronation.

2. **K – Triceps**
   The three heads of the triceps converge onto a common tendon. The muscle is a powerful extensor of the elbow joint.

3. **E – Extensor carpi radialis brevis**
   The extensor carpi radialis longus is attached to the adjacent supracondylar ridge. The extensor carpi radialis longus and brevis are attached distally to the second and third metacarpal bones. They extend the wrist and, with flexor carpi radialis, also abduct the joint.

4. **B – Brachialis**
   The proximal attachment of the brachialis is to the lower anterior surface of the humerus. The muscle is a powerful flexor of the elbow joint.

5. **J – Supinator**
   The proximal attachment of the two heads of the supinator are to the lateral epicondyle of the humerus and the supinator crest of the ulna, adjacent to the trochlear notch. The supinator is a powerful supinator of the forearm.

   The biceps is attached proximally to the scapula, by the long head to the supraglenoid tubercle and by the short head to the tip of the corocoid process. The common tendon is attached to the radial tuberosity. The biceps is a powerful supinator and flexes the elbow most effectively with the forearms supinated.

   Deltoid passes from an extensive attachment on the anterior aspect of the clavicle and the spine of the scapula, to the lateral aspect of the mid-humerus. The deltoid is the main adductor of the shoulder joint.

   The flexor carpi ulnaris has humeral and ulnar heads, bridging over the ulnar nerve; the tendon is attached to the pisiform bone. Flexor carpi ulnaris is a flexor and adductor of the wrist joint.

   Flexor digitorum profundus has an extensive attachment to the anterior aspect of the ulna and adjacent interosseus membrane. Its tendons pass to the base of the distal phalanges of the fingers.

   Flexor pollicis longus is attached proximally to the anterior radius and adjacent interosseus membrane, the tendon passing to the base of the distal phalanx of the thumb. The muscle flexes the metacarpal, phalangeal and interphalangeal joints of the thumb.

   Pronator teres has humeral and ulnar heads that converge, the distal attachment being to the lateral aspect of the mid-radius. The muscle pronates the forearm and is a weak flexor of the elbow.

4. RELATIONSHIPS OF THE UPPER LIMB

1. **H – Radial nerve**
   The radial nerve lies in the radial groove before piercing the lateral intermuscular septum to lie deep to the brachioradialis muscle. It can be damaged by mid-shaft fractures.

2. **J – Ulnar nerve**
   The ulnar nerve then passes deep to the flexor carpi ulnaris, to lie on the flexor digitorum profundus. It is palpable subcutaneously behind the medial epicondyle and can be traumatised at this point.

3. **E – Median nerve**
   In contrast, the ulnar artery passes deep to both heads.

4. **C – Brachial artery**
   The brachial artery lies in the groove between the biceps and brachialis muscles in the arm and divides into the ulnar and radial arteries.

5. G – Radial artery

The radial artery lies on the flexor pollicis longus and pronator quadratus in the forearm before passing lateral to the wrist in the floor of the anatomical snuff box.

5. CUTANEOUS INNERVATION OF THE LOWER LIMB

1. B – Genitofemoral nerve

The genitofemoral nerve supplies the skin over the femoral triangle through its femoral branch. Below this, the anterior and medial aspects of the thigh are supplied by the medial and intermediate cutaneous branches of the femoral nerve.

2. D – Lateral cutaneous nerve of the thigh

The lateral cutaneous nerve of the thigh passes deep to the lateral aspect of the inguinal ligament, piercing the deep fascia 4–5 cm below the anterior superior iliac spine. It divides into anterior and posterior branches, which supply the lateral aspect of the thigh. The nerve can be entrapped within the inguinal ligament, producing a painful syndrome known as 'meralgia paraesthetica'.

3. I – Superficial peroneal (musculocutaneous) nerve

The superficial peroneal nerve is a terminal branch of the common peroneal nerve. Its cutaneous termination supplies the skin over the anterior ankle, dorsum of the foot, and the adjacent sides of the second and third, and third and fourth toes.

4. J – Sural nerve

The sural nerve, with a variable contribution from the sural communicating nerve, supplies the lower lateral part of the back of the leg, the lateral border of the foot and the lateral side of the little toe.

5. A – Deep peroneal (anterior tibial) nerve

The superficial peroneal is a terminal branch of the common peroneal nerve. Its cutaneous distribution is limited to the adjacent sides of the great and second toes.

The posterocutaneous nerve of the thigh supplies the lower buttock and the posterior aspect of the thigh, the popliteal fossa and proximal calf.

The posterior tibial nerve supplies the skin over the sole through the cutaneous branches of its lateral and medial plantar terminal branches. The cutaneous nerves correspond to the distribution of the ulnar and median nerves of the hands, supplying the nail beds as well as the plantar aspects of the toes.

The saphenous nerve is a branch of the femoral nerve. It pierces the deep fascia in the lower medial thigh to pass distally with the great saphenous vein. It is distributed to the skin of the medial side of the leg and foot. The nerve can be damaged during surgery on the great saphenous vein.

6. NERVE SUPPLY OF THE MUSCLES OF THE LOWER LIMB

1. **F – Obturator nerve**
   The obturator nerve also supplies obturator externus and adductor brevis, and occasionally pectineus and adductor magnus, the latter also receiving a contribution from the sciatic nerve, being developmentally a part of the hamstring complex.

2. **G – Sciatic nerve**
   The sciatic nerve usually supplies biceps, semitendinosus, semimembranosus and the ischial part of adductor magnus, before dividing into its tibial and common peroneal components. If there is a high division, biceps receives contributions from both tributaries.

3. **A – Deep peroneal (anterior tibial) nerve**
   The deep peroneal nerve also gives muscular branches to tibialis anterior, extensor digitorum longus and peroneus tertius.

4. **H – Superficial peroneal (musculocutaneous) nerve**
   The superficial peroneal nerve supplies both peroneus longus and brevis.

5. **J – Tibial (posterior tibial) nerve**
   The tibial nerve supplies the muscles of the posterior aspect of the lower leg before dividing into medial and lateral plantar nerves. The muscles it innervates include gastrocnemius, plantaris, soleus, popliteus, flexor digitorum longus and flexor hallucis.

   The common peroneal nerve is one of the terminal divisions of the sciatic nerve and can supply some of the hamstring muscles if the sciatic nerve divides proximally. The nerve divides into deep and superficial peroneal nerves, but has no direct muscular branches. Damage to the nerve adjacent to the neck of the fibula causes foot drop.

   The femoral nerve is the largest branch of the lumbar plexus. In the abdomen, it supplies branches to the iliacus and pectineus; in the thigh, it supplies the sartorius and quadriceps femoris muscles.

   The inferior gluteal nerve supplies gluteus maximus; the medial plantar nerve supplies the adductor hallucis, flexor digitorum brevis, flexor hallucis brevis, and the first lumbrical.

   The sural nerve is sensory and has no muscle innervation.

7. RELATIONSHIPS OF THE LOWER LIMB

1. **E – Great saphenous vein**
   The great saphenous vein is formed on the medial aspect of the dorsum of the foot and passes along the medial aspect of the leg and thigh. After passing through the saphenous opening, it joins the femoral vein. The small saphenous vein passes behind the lateral malleolus and along the middle of the calf to pierce the popliteal fossa and join the popliteal vein.

2. **C – Femoral artery**
The femoral artery is formed at the mid-inguinal point. It passes distally through the femoral triangle and through the subsartorial canal. It becomes the popliteal artery as it passes with its vein through the hiatus in adductor magnus. The femoral nerve lies lateral to the artery as it emerges from under the inguinal ligament.

3. **B – Common peroneal nerve**
The sciatic nerve leaves the pelvis through the greater sciatic notch, and injections into the gluteus maximus muscle must be aimed upwards and laterally to avoid damaging the nerve at this point. It divides into tibial and common peroneal nerves in the mid thigh and these diverge in the popliteal fossa. The common peroneal nerve is palpable and at risk of injury as it crosses the fibula to divide into superficial and deep peroneal nerves, respectively supplying the peroneal and anterior crural muscles. The tibial nerve supplies the superficial and deep muscles of the posterior aspect of the lower leg.

4. **G – Posterior tibial artery**
The popliteal artery passes deep to the heads of the gastrocnemius muscle. The anterior tibial branch passes over the interosseus membrane into the anterior compartment. It becomes the dorsalis pedis as it crosses the ankle joint midway between the two malleoli and is palpable at this site. The dorsalis pedis artery is also palpable as it crosses the tarsus in the direction of the first digital web. The posterior tibial artery gives off the peroneal branch and then passes between the superficial and deep posterior muscles of the calf. It is palpable behind the tibia and over the talus as it passes into the foot.

5. **F – Peroneal artery**
The peroneal artery passes through the lateral compartment of the lower leg. It can become prominent if the anterior or posterior tibial arteries are congenitally small or diseased. It is then palpable anterior to the lateral malleolus.

8. MUSCLE ATTACHMENTS OF THE LOWER LIMB

1. **F – Rectus femoris**
The rectus femoris with the vastus medialis, intermedius and lateralis make up the quadriceps femoris, which is the powerful knee extensor muscle, making up the bulk of the anterior thigh. The other three muscles gain extensive attachments from the shaft of the femur and all four are attached to the patella and thence by the patellar tendon to the tibial tubercle.

2. **A – Adductor longus**
The adductors longus, brevis and magnus gain attachment to the pubic bone, but the adductor magnus, which is developmentally also part of the hamstring muscle group, is also attached to the ischial tuberosity. Distally, the three muscles are attached to the medial side of the femur, the adductor magnus by an extensive expansion down to the adductor tubercle on the medial condyle. These muscles are adductors of the hip joint.

3. **C – Biceps femoris**
The biceps femoris, like the semimembranosus, is attached proximally to the ischial tuberosity. It also has a femoral head. The semimembranosus is attached distally to the medial tibial condyle. The two muscles are powerful knee flexors.

4. **I – Tibialis anterior**
The tibialis anterior has an extensive proximal attachment to the shaft of the tibia and distally is attached to the medial and inferior aspect of the medial cuneiform and adjacent first metatarsal. It dorsiflects the ankle and helps to maintain the medial longitudinal arch of the foot.

5. **D – Peroneus brevis**
The peronei longus and brevis are attached proximally along the lateral aspect of the fibula. Distally, the peroneus longus passes under the foot to be attached to the medial cuneiform and first metatarsal. The muscles evert the foot and the peroneus longus also helps maintain the lateral longitudinal arch of the foot.

The soleus, with the gastrocnemius muscle, forms the prominence of the calf. The soleus has tibial and fibular heads and the two muscles have a common tendo calcaneus. They are powerful plantarflexors of the ankle. Tibialis posterior is attached proximally to the posterior aspect of the tibia and adjacent interosseus membrane. It passes around the medial malleolus to be attached to the tubercle of the navicular bone. The muscle is the main invertor of the foot and assists in plantarflexion.

9. COMPLICATIONS OF FRACTURES

1. **C – Compartment syndrome**
This patient has a supracondylar fracture of the humerus with secondary compartment syndrome. This injury is confined to childhood, when it is quite common. The humeral fracture is just above the condyles and the distal fragment is pushed and tilted backwards. While the great danger of supracondylar fracture is direct primary injury to the brachial artery, when peripheral ischaemia can be immediate and severe, more commonly forearm oedema and an increasing compartment pressure lead to necrosis of muscle and nerve, due to severe ischaemia. The clinical features are those of ischaemia (pain, paraesthesiae, pallor, paralysis and pulselessness) but, commonly, severe pain and swelling are the only features present and the presence of a pulse (as in this case) does not exclude the diagnosis.

2. **G – Non-union**
This patient has a fracture of the scaphoid which has been missed at his first hospital visit because the radiograph appeared normal, as is sometimes be the case in the initial stages of this injury. The fracture has subsequently failed to unite because of continued movement at the fracture line. This might have been prevented by immobilisation of the fracture at the initial visit, when it should have been suspected on the basis of the mechanism of injury and clinical examination. A second radiograph at 2 weeks confirms the fracture in most cases.

3. **F – Nerve injury**
This footballer has a fracture dislocation of the knee, which was reduced in the Emergency Department. This serious injury has a high association with vascular and nerve injuries. In this case there is no vascular injury, but the foot pulses should always be checked. The neurological injury is an injury of the common peroneal nerve. This nerve supplies motor fibres to the anterior and peroneal muscle compartments of the

lower leg (dorsiflexion and eversion of the foot) and sensory fibres to the skin of the lower leg and the dorsum of the foot.

4.   A – Algodystrophy (Sudeck's atrophy)
This patient has a Colles' fracture (transverse fracture of the distal radius with dorsal displacement of the distal fragment) and Sudeck's reflex sympathetic dystrophy. This is an extremely disabling condition in which the hand becomes painful, stiff and hypersensitive, resisting all forms of treatment for months. The condition is usually seen in the hand or the foot, often after relatively trivial injury. With prolonged physiotherapy there is usually steady, albeit slow recovery.

5.   I – Osteoarthritis
The long timescale after the injury with initial recovery suggests this common complication of fractures. Osteoarthritis commonly occurs when fractures disrupt the normal smooth articulation of synovial joints by altering the contour of articulating surfaces (eg intra-articular fractures). The wrist is a common site for such problems, which can have devastating consequences in terms of the patient's occupation (as in this case).

10. UPPER LIMB INJURIES

1.   C – Dislocated shoulder
This patient has a dislocated shoulder. The history of the injury and squaring of the outline of the shoulder is characteristic. The diagnosis is further supported by the finding of neuropraxia of the axillary nerve: this injury is not uncommon and usually recovers spontaneously in a few weeks.

2.   G – Fracture of the shaft of the humerus
This fracture is common in the elderly. The extensive bruising is characteristic. The diagnosis is supported in this case by the finding of wrist drop, which has been caused by a radial nerve injury where it lies in the spiral groove of the humerus. In closed injuries the nerve is seldom divided and the wrist can be splinted while the injury recovers.

3.   I I – Scaphoid fracture
This patient has a scaphoid fracture and avascular necrosis of the scaphoid bone. The injury is caused by a fall onto the dorsiflexed hand. The appearance can be deceptively normal and is sometimes dismissed by patients (and occasionally by clinicians) as a sprained wrist. The classic clinical feature is of fullness and tenderness in the anatomical snuffbox (the depression on the dorsilateral wrist formed by the extensor and abductor tendons to the thumb). If immobilisation is not adequate, the proximal fragment of the scaphoid can necrose and cause persistent pain and weakness of the wrist.

4.   J – Supracondylar fracture of the humerus
This injury is confined to childhood, when it is quite common. The humerus fractures just above the condyles and the distal fragment is pushed and tilted backwards. The great danger of supracondylar fracture is direct primary injury to the brachial artery, leading to immediate and severe peripheral ischaemia, as in this case.

5.   **F – Fracture of the radial head**
     This patient has a fracture of the radial head, as evidenced by the mechanism of injury, presentation and radiological appearance. The fracture line itself is not always obvious if the fracture is undisplaced, but is strongly suggested by the clinical findings, and the finding of an effusion, which is indicated by the displacement of the fat pad. The injury is sometimes associated with a slight long-term decrease in range of movements at the elbow, especially extension.

11. MONOARTHRITIS

1.   **D – Gout**
     This patient has developed an acute episode of gout. This is confirmed by the characteristic appearance of the crystals aspirated from the joint. Acutely, he should be treated with rest and NSAIDs or colchicine. His risk factors, such as alcohol excess, should be addressed. In the long term he should be treated with allopurinol, but this should never be started in the acute attack because it can exacerbate the condition.

2.   **G – Pyrophosphate arthritis**
     This patient has developed pyrophosphate arthropathy or 'pseudogout'. This is a commoner cause of a monoarthritis in the elderly than gout, although they present in a similar manner. This condition is confirmed by the presence of the intra-articular calcification and the characteristic appearance of the crystals under polarised light.

3.   **H – Reiter's syndrome**
     This patient has developed the classic triad of Reiter's syndrome (ie acute arthritis associated with conjunctivitis and a non-specific urethritis). It is an HLA-B27 disorder and is a reactive arthritis associated with sexually transmitted diseases and acute diarrhoeal infections (eg *Chlamydia*, *Campylobacter*, *Shigella* and *Yersinia*).

4.   **B – Charcot's joint**
     This patient has developed a 'Charcot deformity' of the ankle. This arises in weight-bearing joints (mainly the ankle) and is thought to be due to neurovascular changes rather than simply to neurotrauma. The deformity is most commonly associated with chronic sensory neuropathies such as those of diabetes mellitus, syphilis (tabes dorsalis) and syringomyelia.

5.   **I – Staphylococcal arthritis**
     This woman has developed an acute septic arthritis of the shoulder after her intra-articular injection. The most likely causative organisms are streptococcal and staphylococcal species and the empirical antibiotic therapy should include intravenous benzylpenicillin and flucloxacillin. For diagnostic and therapeutic (analgesic) purposes, the shoulder should be aspirated (ensuring an aseptic technique).

12. POLYARTHRITIS

1. **D – Psoriasis**
   This patient has psoriatic arthropathy. This can mimic rheumatoid arthritis in clinical appearance and progression and might only be distinguishable by the presence of psoriatic skin and nail changes. Psoriasis is associated with several patterns of arthropathy, including an asymmetrical arthritis that principally affects the distal interphalangeal joints, arthritis mutilans, an asymmetrical mono- or oligo-arthropathy and sacroiliitis.

2. **C – Osteoarthritis**
   This patient has osteoarthritis of the hands and knee. It is more common in the weight-bearing joints of obese patients but can affect almost any joint. The asymmetrical arthropathy of the distal interphalangeal joints of the hands is associated with Bouchard's and Heberden's nodes affecting the proximal and distal interphalangeal joints, respectively.

3. **A – Behçet's disease**
   This gentleman has an acute exacerbation of his Behçet's disease, an idiopathic disorder caused by inflammation of the venules. It is strongly associated with HLA-B51 and is thought to be triggered by an environmental agent. It is characterised by recurrent episodes of ulceration, particularly of the mouth and genitalia, and uveitis. The arthritis accompanying the acute episodes is usually asymmetrical and predominantly affects the joints of the lower limbs. It is non-erosive and responds to steroid therapy.

4. **J – Systemic lupus erythematosus**
   This patient has SLE, as evidenced by the autoantibodies and the characteristic 'butterfly' rash. The associated arthritis is usually asymmetrical and can affect several joints. It is classically non-erosive but can be associated with chronic deformity, such as 'Z' thumbing (as seen in rheumatoid disease) due to joint capsule and ligament damage.

5. **H – Sjögren's syndrome**
   This woman has developed a secondary Sjögren's syndrome, characterised by rheumatoid arthritis associated with dry mouth (xerostomia) and dry eyes (keratocon-junctivitis sicca). The sicca syndrome is due to T-cell infiltration of the lacrimal and salivary glands. Other affected areas can include the pancreas (causing malab-sorption), the vagina (dyspareunia) and the gastrointestinal tract (oesophagitis, gastritis and constipation).

13. COMPLICATIONS OF RHEUMATOID ARTHRITIS

1. **C – Mononeuritis multiplex**
   This patient has developed a mononeuritis multiplex (ie a neuropathy of two or more nerves that are not anatomically related). In this case she has a left median nerve lesion and a right peroneal nerve lesion. It is caused by a vasculitis of the vasa nervorum. Other neurological disorders associated with rheumatoid arthritis include a peripheral sensory neuropathy, a mixed motor/sensory neuropathy and an entrapment neuropathy.

2.   **E – Pericarditis**
Cardiac involvement in rheumatoid arthritis includes pericarditis, pericardial effusions (rarely causing tamponade) and constrictive pericarditis.

3.   **F – Peripheral sensory neuropathy**
This patient has developed a peripheral sensory neuropathy. This can be as a result of the disease itself or can be caused by several of the drugs used in the treatment of the disease (eg gold).

4.   **I – Scleromalacia**
This patient has scleritis as evidenced by the pattern of the scleral vessel injection and the pain, which is the differentiating feature from episcleritis, which is painless. Scleritis can lead to thinning of the sclera (scleromalacia) and subsequent perforation.

5.   **B – Felty's syndrome**
This man has developed Felty's syndrome, which is the association of rheumatoid disease with splenomegaly and subsequent pancytopenia and recurrent infections. It usually occurs in patients with long-standing disease (>10 years) and can be associated with weight loss, a vasculitic rash and ulceration.

14. DRUGS USED IN RHEUMATOID ARTHRITIS

1.   **I – Prednisolone**
This patient has signs consistent with iatrogenic Cushing's syndrome, caused by her steroid therapy. It is difficult to avoid this complication in long-term treatment but often 'steroid-sparing' agents such as azathioprine are used in attempt to lower the dosage/duration of steroids employed. All patients on long-term steroid therapy need to carry a steroid card to notify medical staff and should be placed on bone-sparing agents such as a bisphosphonate, to avoid their osteoporotic side-effects.

2.   **D – Diclofenac**
Recently, two cyclo-oxygenase (COX) receptors have been identified, COX-1 and COX-2. It is thought that the inhibition of COX-1 receptors mediates the unwanted gastrointestinal side-effects and COX-2 inhibition mediates the anti-inflammatory effects. It was hoped that the development of newer NSAIDs, such as rofecoxib and celecoxib (which are more selective against COX-2) would reduce the gastrointestinal side-effects, but recent reviews have not confirmed their promise. The COX index is a ratio of a NSAID's activity against COX-1/COX-2, with the more traditional NSAIDs having a ratio above 1 (ie they inhibit COX-1 more than COX-2 receptors).

3.   **G – Hydroxychloroquine**
This patient has been started on hydroxychloroquine. Many of the disease-modifying agents (disease-modifying agents of rheumatoid disease, or DMARDs) have similar side-effects, including skin rashes, bone marrow suppression and other haematological side-effects, and liver and renal effects. The antimalarial drugs such as hydroxychloroquine also cause eye problems but the retinopathy is rare at normal therapeutic doses. This group of drugs should only be prescribed by rheumatologists with access to frequent blood monitoring.

4. **E – D-Penicillamine**
    This patient has developed a 'lupus-like' syndrome associated with penicillamine. Other drugs that cause this rare side-effect include hydralazine, isoniazid, phenytoin and procainamide, as well as penicillin and sulphonamides. The drug-induced syndrome commonly affects the lungs but rarely involves the kidneys. The syndrome is characterised by high titres of antinuclear antibody (ANA) but normal double binding. These immune markers disappear with withdrawal of the drug but will reappear with its re-introduction.

5. **F – Gold**
    This patient has developed bone marrow suppression, leading to anaemia, agranulocytosis (and infection) and a purpuric rash. This can be secondary to treatment with several of the DMARDs but only gold is given by weekly injection. When prescribing any new medication, patients must be warned of potential side-effects and what to do if they occur.

15. PREDISPOSING FACTORS TO OSTEOARTHROPATHIES

1. **F – Obesity**
    This woman's BMI is 35.8 kg/m², which indicates that she is obese (ie the BMI is >28). Obesity is one of the commonest underlying exacerbating problems for patients with osteoarthritis, and weight loss often helps symptoms.

2. **H – Paget's bone disease**
    The radiological appearances described here and the normal serum calcium and phosphate with a raised alkaline phosphatase are characteristic of Paget's bone disease. Paget's bone disease can cause bony pain due to secondary osteoarthritis or to pathological fractures.

3. **B – Avascular necrosis**
    Avascular necrosis is a recognised complication of sickle-cell disease and can cause secondary osteoarthritis. Other causes of avascular necrosis include trauma and fractures, steroid therapy and radiotherapy.

4. **D – Ehlers–Danlos syndrome**
    This man has a relatively benign form of the Ehlers–Danlos syndrome. This is a relatively rare disorder with variable modes of inheritance. Nine variations of the syndrome have now been defined, all associated with abnormal collagen synthesis. Patients have varying degrees of joint hyperextensibility, skin extensibility and fragility, and some have ocular problems.

16. SERONEGATIVE SPONDOARTHROPATHIES

1. **E – Psoriasis**
   This patient has psoriasis-associated arthropathy – in this case the 'telescoping' deformity of the fingers suggests arthritis mutilans.

2. **B – Ankylosing spondylitis**
   This patient has ankylosing spondylitis with associated apical fibrosis of the lungs. The fibrosis is rare, occurring in approximately 1% of cases, but respiratory problems secondary to the severe kyphosis are common. Other associations include sacroiliitis (which is almost universal); peripheral joint involvement (particularly of the lower limbs), which occurs in 30–40% of cases; anterior uveitis; and aortitis leading to aortic regurgitation. Around 80–95% of cases are associated with the presence of HLA-B27.

3. **G – Reiter's syndrome**
   This patient has developed a Reiter's syndrome with associated heel pain. This might be due to Achilles' tendonitis or plantar fascitis.

4. **D – Enteropathic synovitis**
   This man has inflammatory bowel disease associated with enteropathic synovitis. The activity of this non-erosive arthropathy is related to the relapses and remissions of the bowel disease. It is commonly associated with the other extragastrointestinal complications, including anterior uveitis, erythema nodosum, pyoderma gangrenosum and finger clubbing. A similar disorder can also occur after gastrointestinal bypass surgery.

5. **H – Whipple's disease**
   This man has developed Whipple's disease, as evidenced by his presentation and the characteristic PAS-positive macrophages in his biopsy specimens. The causative organism has now been identified, a Gram-positive bacillus called *Tropheryma whippelii*. The disease responds to antibiotic treatment with penicillin, erythromycin or tetracycline.

17. REITER'S SYNDROME

1. **C, D, E – Arthritis, circinate balanitis and conjunctivitis**

2. **C, E, F, J – Arthritis, conjunctivitis, keratoderma blennorrhagicum and urethritis**

3. **B, C, I – Anterior uveitis, arthritis and plantar fasciitis**

4. **A, I – Achilles' tendonitis and plantar fasciitis**
   Reiter's syndrome is the triad of acute arthritis (usually of a lower limb joint), conjunctivitis and urethritis. It is strongly associated with HLA-B27. The syndrome develops as a result of exposure to a 'trigger' infection, either gastrointestinal or a sexually transmitted infection. Causative organisms include *Chlamydia*, *Salmonella*, *Yersinia* and *Campylobacter*. The classic triad can be associated with fever, malaise and several systemic complications, including:

   - Eyes: anterior uveitis (usually mild) – can pre-date acute episodes of the triad
   - Oral ulceration

- Circinate balanitis: ulceration of the glans of the penis – often painless
- Keratoderma blennorrhagicum: this rash affects the soles and, less commonly, the palms. It rarely occurs unless the complete triad is present
- Achilles' tendonitis and plantar fascitis: these can lead to calcaneal erosions in persisting disease.

The acute arthritis is treated with rest, physiotherapy and NSAIDs. Large effusions might need to be aspirated. The aspirate is sterile. The underlying infection also needs to be treated.

18. VASCULITIDES

1. **H – Wegener's granulomatosis**
   Wegener's granulomatosis is a small-vessel necrotising vasculitis that is characterised by upper and lower respiratory tract involvement, associated with a renal vasculitis. The characteristic immune marker is c-ANCA; the principal antigen in the cytoplasm has now been identified as being proteinase 3. Cyclophosphamide has revolutionised the treatment of this disorder which until 20 years ago was invariably fatal.

2. **F – Polyarteritis nodosa**
   Polyarteritis nodosa (PAN) is a medium-vessel, non-granulomatous vasculitis that is characterised by aneurysm formation in affected tissues. It can affect the kidneys, liver, heart, gastrointestinal tract, skin and even the cerebral circulation. There are no known immune markers characterising the condition but a significant minority of affected patients are hepatitis B surface antigen (HBsAg) positive. The significance of this anti-genaemia is as yet unknown.

3. **B – Giant-cell arteritis**
   This patient has the classic symptoms of temporal arteritis, which can form part of a generalised giant-cell arteritis. This vasculitis forms part of a spectrum with polymyalgia rheumatica and is characterised by an ESR greater than 100 mm/h. The generalised disorder can be associated with myocardial, cerebral, mesenteric or limb ischaemia. The diagnosis should be confirmed by arterial biopsy but steroids should be started as soon as the diagnosis is suspected in order to protect against further complications.

4. **A – Churg–Strauss syndrome**
   Churg–Strauss syndrome can be regarded as a variant of polyarteritis nodosa. Unlike PAN, however, it is a small-vessel necrotising granulomatous disease that principally affects the lungs. It can present in a similar fashion to asthma and can be associated with a peripheral eosinophilia. There are no characteristic immune markers but occasionally perinuclar ANCA (p-ANCA) titres are raised.

5. **C – Henoch–Schönlein purpura**
   Henoch–Schönlein purpura is a small-vessel vasculitis that can occur at any age. It is characterised by a rapidly coalescing purpuric rash that usually affects the lower limbs and buttocks. It can be associated with a flitting arthritis, particularly of the lower limbs, and a glomerulonephritis. IgA titres are raised in approximately 50% of patients.

19. CHRONDROCALCINOSIS

Chondrocalcinosis is the intra-articular deposition of calcium.

1. **H – Pyrophosphate arthropathy**
    This patient has developed a pyrophosphate arthropathy or 'pseudogout'. This condition is probably the commonest cause of chondrocalcinosis. It commonly presents in older age as a monoarthropathy and can mimic gout. The aspirate is characterised by crystals that are positively birefringent under polarised light. The condition responds to treatment with NSAIDs.

2. **C – Haemochromatosis**
    This alcohol abuser has developed haemochromatosis. Approximately 25% of patients with the primary condition have a history of alcohol excess, although the alcohol probably acts as an accelerating agent, rather than as the principal cause. The 'unexpected suntan' is due to melanin deposition in the skin and not haemosiderin. She has also developed diabetes mellitus due to pancreatic involvement and cirrhosis. Approximately 30% of patients will develop primary hepatocellular carcinoma.

3. **D – Hyperparathyroidism**
    Hyperparathyroidism classically presents with 'moans (depression), groans (abdominal pains), bones (bony pains), and (renal) stones'. The associated hypercalcaemia can be asymptomatic and only discovered incidentally or as a result of a diagnosis of chondrocalcinosis on a radiograph.

4. **B – Gout**
    This patient has severe, tophaceous gout, causing the exuding nodules. This arthropathy is treated with NSAIDs or colchicine in the first instance and prophylaxis with allopurinol should be added once the acute episode has resolved.

5. **F – Hypothyroidism**
    This woman has a classic presentation of hypothyroidism. Clues in the blood tests include the macrocytosis and the hyponatraemia, which is thought to be due to a syndrome of inappropriate antidiuretic hormone secretion (SIADH).

20. RAISED ESR

1. **A – Carcinomatosis**
    This patient has carcinomatosis, as evidenced by the deranged LFTs, the cannon-ball metastases on the chest radiograph and the hypercalcaemia. The hyponatraemia could be secondary to a SIADH caused by the lung metastases or possibly the cerebral metastases.

2. **H – Toxic shock syndrome**
    This young woman has developed a toxic shock syndrome. This is usually secondary to a staphylococcal infection but can also occur with other organisms such as *Streptococcus*. The exotoxin (toxic shock syndrome toxin-1, or TSST-1) secreted by such organisms causes severe systemic problems, including multiorgan failure, cardiovascular collapse and disseminated intravascular coagulation (DIC). In young women presenting with this clinical picture, a retained tampon should be excluded. Prompt

antibiotic therapy and support with fluids and inotropes in a high-dependency or intensive-care unit is necessary.

3. **C – Multiple myeloma**
This man has developed multiple myeloma, as evidenced by the hypercalcaemia, the Bence Jones proteinuria and the monoclonal gammopathy.

4. **D – Polymyalgia rheumatica**
This patient has polymyalgia rheumatica, which can be regarded as one end of a spectrum, with giant-cell arteritis at the other extreme. It is rare before the age of 50 and patients often present with non-specific pains around the shoulders and pelvic girdle. The muscles can be tender and stiff but there is not usually associated weakness. Treatment is with oral steroids.

5. **F – Staphylococcal endocarditis**
This intravenous drug abuser has developed a staphylococcal endocarditis. This is a relatively malignant condition and often presents with cardiac failure and systemic features of sepsis. The affected valve often becomes rapidly regurgitant and will invariably require surgical replacement.

In principal, an ESR raised to >100 mm/h is caused by one of four things:
1. Vasculitis – giant-cell arteritis, Wegener's granulomatosis.
2. Disseminated or severe sepsis – tuberculosis, toxic shock, endocarditis.
3. Multiple myeloma, other haematological malignancies, carcinomatosis.
4. Polymyalgia rheumatica (although this is only responsible for 2% of all patients with an ESR > 100 mm/h).

21. AUTOANTIBODIES

1. **C – Anti-dsDNA**
This young woman has developed SLE, characterised by the malar rash associated with pancytopenia and renal impairment. Recently, SLE has been subdivided into several distinct syndromes, each characterised by an autoantibody. This complicates an already difficult multisystem disorder but some basic facts remain.

SLE is a multisystem, autoimmune disorder which characteristically affects women of childbearing age. It is a chronic, relapsing disorder but can resolve spontaneously or eventually burn itself out. The principal cause of disease-related mortality is the renal disease. Common effects include:

- Rheumatological – arthralgia, non-erosive arthritis (the arthritis can be associated with deformity, due to chronic tendonitis and contractures)
- Renal – glomerulonephritis, tubular disorders
- Respiratory – pleurisy, atelectasis
- Cardiac – pancarditis, (ie peri/myo/endocarditis)
- Haematological – pancytopenia, splenomegaly, lymphadenopathy
- Dermatological – photosensitivity, malar rash, ulceration, alopecia, Raynaud's phenomenon
- Vasculitis – can lead to neuropathy and nephropathy.

The mainstay of treatment remains steroids, with immunosuppressive agents such as azathioprine used as a steroid-sparing agent and cyclophosphamide reserved for steroid-resistant cases.

2. **B – Anticentromere**

Systemic sclerosis is another disorder which has been redefined in the light of greater immunological and molecular understanding. The disease can be seen as a spectrum, ranging from Raynaud's phenomenon and positive autoantibodies to a diffuse systemic disease.

The classic CREST syndrome (**c**alcinosis, **R**aynaud's, o**e**sophageal dysmotility, **s**clerodactyly and **t**elangiectasia) is now called 'limited cutaneous systemic sclerosis'. It is characterised by early development of Raynaud's, often pre-dating the other features by many years. Skin changes then develop and over the next 10 years the other features, including pulmonary disease, begin to manifest. The immune marker of this disease is the anticentromere antibody.

Diffuse cutaneous systemic sclerosis can begin in a similar manner to the limited form, but the skin changes often develop earlier and are associated with earlier pulmonary and renal disease. These are accompanied by cardiac and upper and lower gastrointestinal tract involvement. This condition is characterised by the presence of the anti-Scl-70 antibody, although it is only present in approximately 30% of cases.

Scleroderma sine scleroderma represents a further division and is characterised by Raynaud's with any of the other features, but no skin changes. Either of the autoantibodies can be present in this condition.

3. **D – Anti-Jo-1**

This man has developed dermatomyositis, which is often associated with underlying malignancy in mid- to late life. This condition is characterised by the Anti-Jo-1 antibody. The rash around the eyes is characteristic and is described as heliotropic; it can also occur over the dorsum of the fingers (knuckles) and the extensor surfaces of the knees and elbows.

4. **I – c-ANCA**

This man has the classi triad of Wegener's granulomatosis (ie renal impairment associated with both upper and lower respiratory involvement). The condition is characterised by the c-ANCA autoantibody, although, rarely, this can also occur in other vasculitic conditions. The p-ANCA autoantibody was initially thought to characterise microscopic polyangiitis but more recent work has shown that it is seen in a host of conditions, including PAN, immune hepatitis, inflammatory bowel disease and sclerosing cholangitis.

5. **A – Anticardiolipin**

This patient has an antiphospholipid syndrome, characterised by miscarriages and arterial and venous thromboses. The syndrome can be primary or secondary and is marked by autoantibodies reacting against various phospholipids, including cardiolipin. Anticardiolipin antibodies are often associated with the lupus syndrome. Patients with this condition should be placed on long-term anticoagulation. Such antibodies can also occur in acute infections, when they are usually transient and do not require further treatment.

NB: Anti-Ro and Anti-La autoantibodies characterise Sjögren's syndrome but can occur in several of the syndromes in SLE. Anti-RNP is seen in SLE syndromes with overlap features such as Raynaud's phenomenon or myositis.

22. RAYNAUD'S PHENOMENON

Raynaud's phenomenon can be a primary or secondary condition. The primary disorder is known as 'Raynaud's disease' and is an idiopathic condition with no associated autoantibodies. The disease is due to an exaggerated vascular response to cold weather and causes characteristic, painful colour changes of the digits. The fingers and toes blanch on exposure to cold; on reheating, the white digits become blue and finally a hyperaemic red, associated with pain. Secondary Raynaud's phenomenon can develop several years prior to clinical expression of an underlying condition, and patients should have a full autoantibody screen when they present with this condition. The phenomenon also occurs as a result of damage to small vessels caused by trauma of vibrating tools, cold injury and toxins such as ergot and lead. Large-vessel and proximal arterial disease can reduce distal pressure, making the digital vessels more sensitive to the cold.

1. **G – Sjögren's syndrome**
    This patient has Sjögren's syndrome, probably secondary to rheumatoid arthritis. The disorder is characterised by infiltration of exocrine glands by lymphocytes, leading to symptoms such as xerostomia (dry mouth) and keratoconjunctivitis (dry eyes). This patient might have Anti-Ro and Anti-La antibodies, as well as antinuclear antibody (ANA) and rheumatoid factor.

2. **A – Cervical rib**
    This young man has a cervical rib, which is causing his Raynaud's. A cervical rib can cause a thoracic outlet syndrome, comprising vascular and neurological deficits. The rib might be apparent on a chest radiograph or on thoracic outlet views. A minority of these patients have symptoms due to fibrous bands, though these are not demonstrable on chest radiography.

3. **E – Hypothyroidism**
    This patient has signs and symptoms suggestive of hypothyroidism. The early clubbing is in fact thyroid acropachy and the rash over the shins is pre-tibial myxoedema. These are two of the three features of Graves' triad, the third being Graves' eye disease (Graves' orbitopathy). Classically, Graves' thyroid disease is associated with thyrotoxicosis but patients can be clinically and biochemically hypothyroid, euthyroid or hyperthyroid.

4. **I – Systemic sclerosis**
    This patient has features suggestive of limited cutaneous systemic sclerosis (see previous theme). Raynaud's is a common feature of all aspects of systemic sclerosis. A pre-scleroderma condition is recognised, with Raynaud's and positive antibodies but few other features of the disease.

5. **H – SLE**
    This patient has a photosensitive rash with Raynaud's, arthralgia and myositis. The presence of ANA suggests a lupus syndrome.

23. BONE PROFILE ABNORMALITIES

1. **B – Chronic renal failure**
    This patient has acute on chronic renal failure. The odd skin discoloration is due to his chronic uraemia. He has a pericardial rub, suggestive of a uraemic pericarditis, and signs of fluid overload. His hyperkalaemia suggests an acute decompensation but the anaemia, hypocalcaemia and hyperphosphataemia suggest a chronic problem. The abnormalities of calcium and vitamin D metabolism in chronic renal failure lead initially to hypocalcaemia and hypophosphataemia, which in turn causes a secondary hyperparathyroidism and, eventually, tertiary hyperparathyroidism. The resulting bone changes are known as 'renal osteodystrophy'.

2. **G – Paget's bone disease**
    The normal calcium and phosphate levels associated with the raised alkaline phosphatase and characteristic radiological changes are suggestive of Paget's bone disease. This is a relatively common disorder of older age and presents with immobility, bone pain, fractures and bone deformity. A rare complication of this disorder is osteosarcoma, which occur in <1% of patients. Hypercalcaemia in association with Paget's bone disease can occur due to chronic immobility or, more commonly, malignant disease.

3. **F – Osteomalacia**
    This patient has developed osteomalacia, as evidenced by her hypocalcaemia (the corrected calcium is often low-normal), hypophosphataemia and raised alkaline phosphatase. This commonly presents with non-specific symptoms, particularly myalgia and pelvic and shoulder girdle weakness. It is common in patients with poor vitamin D intake, poor sunlight exposure and malabsorption. Looser's zones might be evident on radiographs, and these are pathognomonic of osteomalacia, representing incompletely healed stress fractures.

4. **I – Parathyroid hormone-related polypeptide**
    Hypercalcaemia is usually a late presentation of malignant tumours and is most commonly associated with bony metastases. Rarely, however, lung tumours secrete a parathyroid hormone (PTH-)like polypeptide, which can also cause hypercalcaemia. This man also has hyponatraemia, which is probably due to SIADH. Hypercalcaemia of malignancy should be treated with hydration (intravenous fluids are often required) and intravenous pamidronate.

5. **E – Multiple myeloma**
    This man has developed hypercalcaemia associated with multiple myeloma. He also has renal impairment and bone marrow failure, as evidenced by the pancytopenia. He has also developed hepatosplenomegaly with deranged LFTs. He will require intravenous pamidronate, renal replacement therapy and supportive blood transfusions.

24. PROXIMAL MYOPATHY

1. **J – Thyrotoxicosis**

   This patient has developed thyrotoxicosis, as evidenced by her weight loss, resting tachycardia and proximal myopathy. Other clinical signs can include palmar erythema, lid lag (on eye examination) and a thyroid bruit. Endocrine disorders such as thyrotoxicosis, acromegaly, Cushing's disease, diabetes mellitus and osteomalacia are commonly associated with proximal myopathy and weakness.

2. **G – Motor neurone disease**

   This man has developed motor neurone disease. The weakness can be asymmetrical, global, proximal or distal, and is associated with wasting and fasciculation. There are commonly mixed upper and lower motor neurone signs but these are NOT associated with sensory loss, cerebellar or eye signs. The nasal regurgitation of food is common with bulbar/pseudobulbar problems.

3. **A – Acromegaly**

   This patient has acromegaly. This disorder is associated with a growth hormone-secreting tumour of the pituitary gland. Patients present with local features of tumour enlargement, including headache and visual field loss. The classic field loss is bitemporal hemianopia but almost any field deficit is possible. The visual loss is due to compression of the optic chiasma by the expanding tumour. Systemic features include changing facial features, including frontal bossing, coarsening of the facial features and increased interdental separation. The hands and feet enlarge, causing ill-fitting shoes, gloves and rings, and there can be hypertension and diabetes mellitus.

4. **C – Cushing's disease**

   This patient has quite florid features of Cushing's disease, (the pituitary-dependent disease, as opposed to Cushing's syndrome, which is due to extrapituitary causes). The centripetal obesity is associated with proximal myopathy, diabetes mellitus, abdominal striae (which are violaceous) and local features of a pituitary tumour. Treatment might include neurosurgical excision, through a transnasal or a transfrontal approach, which can be combined with radiotherapy.

5. **B – Alcoholic myopathy**

   This patient has features of chronic liver disease, including clubbing of the nails, Dupuytren's contracture and spider naevi. He has now developed an alcoholic myopathy, which can involve the myocardium, leading to cardiac failure. The blood tests show a macrocytosis, thrombocytopenia, hyponatraemia, low urea and deranged LFTs, all indicating alcohol excess.

ANSWERS TO CHAPTER – ENDOCRINE, BREAST, DERMATOLOGY 4

1. HYPOTHALAMIC AND PITUITARY DISEASE

1. J – Sheehan's syndrome
'Sheehan's syndrome' is the term used to describe infarction of the pituitary gland following post-partum haemorrhage. Modern obstetric care has resulted in this becoming a rare disorder in the developed world. It causes symptoms of panhypopituitarism, including failure of lactation (hypoprolactinaemia), secondary amenorrhoea (hypogonadism), fatigue (hypocortisolaemia) and cold intolerance (hypothyroidism), although it can occasionally present acutely with an addisonian crisis. Treatment is with full anterior pituitary hormone replacement.

2. H – Nelson's syndrome
'Nelson's syndrome' is the term used to describe hyperpigmentation and enlargement of a corticotroph adenoma occurring as a late complication of pituitary Cushing's disease that has been treated by bilateral adrenalectomy. It is thought to be caused by removal of negative feedback, in the form of hypercortisolaemia, unmasking aggressive potential in the pituitary tumour. The hyperpigmentation, which affects the mouth as well as the skin, is driven by excessive levels of adrenocorticotrophic hormone (ACTH) and its precursors, as in Addison's disease. The incidence of Nelson's syndrome is reduced by administration of pituitary radiotherapy soon after adrenalectomy.

3. B – Cranial diabetes insipidus
Cranial diabetes insipidus is caused by a deficiency of secretion of antidiuretic hormone (ADH, also known as 'arginine vasopressin') by the posterior pituitary. It is a common complication of pituitary and hypothalamic surgery and also occurs after basal skull fracture, which often results in trauma to the pituitary stalk. Biochemically, it can be demonstrated by an elevated serum osmolality with an inappropriately low urine osmolality, which corrects following administration of desmopressin (des-amino-D-arginine vasopressin or DDAVP), an artificial ADH analogue.

4. F – Lactotroph pituitary macroadenoma
Moderate elevation of serum prolactin (up to 2000 mU/l) can be caused by lactotroph pituitary microadenomas (defined as tumours with a diameter <10 mm that are confined to the pituitary fossa), by dopamine receptor-antagonist medications or by interruption of dopamine-mediated inhibition of prolactin release by pituitary, hypothalamic or other suprasellar lesions, including non-lactotroph pituitary macroadenomas. Gross hyperprolactinaemia, as in this case, occurs as a result of secretion of prolactin by a lactotroph pituitary macroadenoma. Hyperprolactinaemia causes impotence in men, oligo- or amenorrhoea in women, and reduced libido, infertility and galactorrhoea in both sexes. In addition, macroadenomas have local pressure effects, including visual field loss, headache and hypopituitarism.

5.   E – Kallmann's syndrome

Kallmann's syndrome, or isolated hypogonadotrophic hypogonadism, is caused by the failure of development of the hypothalamic neurones, which secrete gonadotrophin-releasing hormone (GnRH). Embryologically, these neurones are derived from olfactory epithelium. Patients with Kallmann's syndrome are characteristically anosmic or hyposmic (lacking a sense of smell) and also frequently demonstrate colour-blindness and have midline facial developmental defects such as cleft lip and palate. Treatment in both sexes is aimed primarily at initiating the development of secondary sexual charac-teristics. Fertility is made possible subsequently with the aid of gonadotrophin prepara-tions or pulsed GnRH.

2.   DISORDERS OF THE HYPOTHALAMO-PITUITARY-ADRENAL AXIS

1.   A – Addison's disease

Thomas Addison's description was of adrenal insufficiency caused by tuberculous destruction of the adrenal glands. The term 'Addison's disease' is now used to describe any form of primary hypoadrenalism, the most common modern cause being autoimmune adrenalitis. This form of illness is commoner in women and is associated with other organ-specific autoimmune diseases, including pernicious anaemia, primary hypothyroidism and type 1 diabetes mellitus. The presentation can be acute and precipitated by other illness, with cardiovascular collapse, or insidious, with weight loss, fatigue, depression and hyperpigmentation. The serum biochemistry clas-sically shows hyponatraemia, hyperkalaemia and uraemia. The plasma ACTH is high. A short Synacthen® (synthetic ACTH) test demonstrates failure of cortisol secretion. Treatment is with glucocorticoid and mineralocorticoid replacement. The patient should carry a steroid card and an intramuscular hydrocortisone emergency pack.

2.   C – Adrenal carcinoma

The elevated cortisol and undetectable ACTH in this case point to autonomous adrenal secretion of cortisol, which can be due either to an adrenal adenoma or to an adrenal carcinoma. The short history of onset and extreme virilisation are character-istic of adrenal carcinoma. Adrenal carcinomas are usually large (diameter >4 cm) at presentation, grow rapidly and metastasise early. Treatment is by surgical excision, followed by oral treatment with Mitotane®, a toxic adrenolytic agent. The prognosis is usually poor.

3.   F – Ectopic adrenocorticotrophic hormone (ACTH) secretion

Cushing's syndrome caused by ectopic ACTH secretion usually has a rapid onset. Weight gain can occur if the source is a tiny bronchial carcinoid tumour, but cachexia and hypokalaemic alkalosis might be the presenting features if a small-cell bronchial carcinoma is the cause. Plasma ACTH levels are usually very high (>400 ng/l) and there is failure of serum cortisol suppression on high-dose dexamethasone and failure of serum cortisol response to corticotrophin-releasing hormone (CRH). If chest radiograhy and fine-cut CT chest fail to demonstrate a likely source, whole-body venous catheter sampling for ACTH might be necessary.

4. **E – Cushing's disease**
    Cushing's syndrome is characterised by failure of serum cortisol to suppress on low-dose dexamethasone (0.5 mg 6-hourly for 48 hours), loss of diurnal variation in cortisol secretion, and loss of cortisol response to an insulin tolerance test. Patients with pituitary Cushing's disease show suppression of serum cortisol on high-dose dexamethasone (2 mg 6-hourly for 48 hours) and have an exaggerated cortisol response to CRH. In such patients, MRI pituitary and inferior petrosal sinus venous catheter sampling are used to demonstrate the presence of a pituitary adenoma and to localise it prior to trans-sphenoidal surgery. If surgery is successful, serum cortisol becomes undetectable post-operatively due to the long-standing suppression of normal corticotroph cells in the pituitary. Glucocorticoid replacement is therefore necessary initially, and is withdrawn periodically during follow-up to assess the recovery of the hypothalamo-pituitary-adrenal axis.

5. **I – Pseudo-Cushing's syndrome**
    Pseudo-Cushing's syndrome results in failure of suppression of serum cortisol on low-dose dexamethasone in association with the characteristic body habitus of Cushing's syndrome. Elevated MCV and serum γ-glutamyltransferase (γGT) can provide clues to the diagnosis. A serum ethanol level in the Out-patients' Department and 1 hour after in-patient visiting has finished can also be useful. Fortunately, the response to the low-dose dexamethasone suppression test normalises rapidly on cessation of drinking.

3. THYROID DISEASE

1. **F – Multinodular goitre**
    Although the appearance is that of a solitary thyroid nodule, the commonest cause of this clinical condition is a single prominent nodule within a multinodular gland. The nodule could nevertheless be a carcinoma, but the finding of increased thyroid function is extremely rare in such cases, although this can occur in multinodular goitre due to the development of autonomous hyperfunctioning nodules – a condition known as 'Plummer's syndrome'.

2. **A – Anaplastic carcinoma**
    This patient has an anaplastic carcinoma of the thyroid. This is a relatively uncommon tumor that occurs in the elderly. The tumour is locally invasive, typically causing recurrent laryngeal nerve palsy and hoarseness and stridor (eventually progressing to asphyxia) because of direct airway invasion. The tumour metastasises early to locoregional lymph nodes and thence to distant sites. It has one of the worst prognoses of any cancer.

3. **C – Graves' disease**
    This patient has Graves' disease, as evidenced by the history of symptoms that suggest thyrotoxicosis, and the thyroid function tests that confirm it. The gland itself is diffusely and smoothly enlarged, though usually only slightly. The hypervascularity might be audible as a bruit. The disease is caused by thyroid-stimulating immunoglobulins that are detectable (where this assay is available) in 90% of cases.

4. **H – Simple colloid goitre**

    This patient has a simple colloid goitre, as evidenced by the clinical findings and the normal thyroid function. Such goitres occur worldwide as a result of iodine deficiency, but also commonly occur during puberty and pregnancy, when the demand for thyroxine is increased and the gland produces more colloid under the stimulus of thyroid-stimulating hormone (TSH), which is released in response to low thyroxine levels in an attempt to increase the thyroxine (hence the finding of a normal T_4 and raised TSH).

5. **E – Medullary thyroid carcinoma**

    The diagnosis is made indirectly on the basis of the biochemical and radiological findings, which provide evidence of the presence of a phaeochromocytoma (raised urinary catecholamines and adrenal mass, hence the hypertensive presentation) and parathyroid hyperplasia (hypercalcaemia secondary to hyperparathyroidism). The association of medullary thyroid carcinoma, phaeochromocytoma and parathyroid hyperplasia is well recognized as the multiple endocrine neoplasia syndrome (MEN) type II. The tumours are rarely palpable within the thyroid gland itself.

4. HYPERGLYCAEMIA

1. **C – Chronic pancreatitis**

    Both endocrine and exocrine functions of the pancreas are affected by chronic pancreatitis. Exocrine dysfunction causes malabsorption, resulting in steatorrhoea and weight loss, while the endocrine dysfunction causes diabetes mellitus. Initial investigations include plain abdominal radiography, looking for speckled calcification of the pancreas, and abdominal ultrasound, looking for pancreatic duct dilatation, pseudo-cysts and ascites. The most common cause of chronic pancreatitis is alcohol abuse.

2. **A – Acromegaly**

    Acromegaly is almost invariably caused by a pituitary adenoma that is secreting growth hormone. Overgrowth of soft tissue and bone causes the characteristic coarse facial features and enlargement of the hands and feet and also predisposes to cardiomegaly, obstructive sleep apnoea and colorectal carcinoma. Local effects of the expanding pituitary tumour include headache, bitemporal hemianopia, resulting from compression of the optic chiasm, and hypopituitarism, resulting from compression normal pituitary tissue. Compression of the pituitary stalk causes hypersecretion of prolactin as a result of a reduction in dopamine-mediated inhibition. Growth hormone excess causes insulin resistance, and this progresses to frank diabetes mellitus in about 20% of patients.

3. **J – Type 1 diabetes mellitus**

    Type 1 diabetes mellitus presents most commonly in children and adolescents. It is characterised by autoimmune-mediated destruction of pancreatic islet β-cells, resulting in total loss of insulin secretion. This is in contrast to type 2 diabetes mellitus, in which insulin resistance leads initially to hyperinsulinaemia, followed by a prolonged and gradual deterioration in β-cell function. The presentation of type 1 diabetes mellitus is with a short history of polyuria, polydipsia, weight loss and lethargy. If the diagnosis is made early enough, subcutaneous insulin treatment can be introduced without admission to hospital. However, if the diagnosis is delayed, ketoacidosis develops, resulting in Kussmaul respiration, reduced conscious level and, eventually, death. Diabetic ketoacidosis is a medical emergency that requires urgent treatment with intravenous insulin and fluid replacement.

4. **G – Haemochromatosis**
Haemochromatosis is an autosomal recessive disease in which disordered regulation of iron stores results in iron deposition throughout the body. Complications include diabetes mellitus, hepatic cirrhosis and hepatocellular carcinoma, cardiomyopathy, arthropathy secondary to chondrocalcinosis, and primary and secondary hypogonadism. Melanin deposition in the skin results in a suntanned appearance. Treatment is with repeated venesection, which prevents new complications arising but does not reverse the diabetes, chondrocalcinosis or gonadal atrophy.

5. **D – Cushing's disease**
Cushing's syndrome results from prolonged, inappropriate exposure to glucocorticoids. The commonest cause is chronic use of steroid medication but the rare, endogenous causes include autonomous adrenal secretion by an adrenal tumour, ectopic ACTH secretion by a neuroendocrine-derived tumour, and Cushing's disease, where ACTH is secreted by a pituitary tumour. The complications of Cushing's syndrome include diabetes mellitus, cardiovascular disease, osteoporosis and infection.

5. COMPLICATIONS OF DIABETES

1. **H – Peripheral sensory neuropathy**
Distal symmetrical sensory polyneuropathy is a common complication of long-standing diabetes. Patients lose vibration, pain and temperature sensation in a 'glove and stocking' distribution. Later, proprioception can be lost, which makes balance difficult in the absence of visual information. When perception of pain is impaired, trauma to the extremities can go unnoticed, predisposing to ulcer formation and Charcot neuropathic arthropathy (painless joint destruction).

2. **A – Amyotrophy**
Diabetic amyotrophy is a painful wasting process which usually affects the quadriceps muscles in one limb only. The pathogenesis is not fully understood but it generally occurs in the context of poor glycaemic control and can resolve once the blood glucose is better managed.

3. **G – Mononeuritis multiplex**
'Mononeuritis multiplex' is the term used for a neuropathy affecting more than one peripheral nerve in isolation. The defect can be motor, sensory or a combination of both and, although recovery is the rule, this is often only partial.

4. **D – Diabetic nephropathy**
Diabetic nephropathy is the most common cause of death in patients with type 1 diabetes mellitus. In its earliest stage, small amounts of albumin are excreted into the urine at levels too low to be detected by standard urinalysis dipsticks ('microalbuminuria'). As the tubular defect worsens, the amount of protein loss increases, hypertension develops, the glomerular filtration rate falls and the patient progresses inexorably towards end-stage renal failure. Recently published trials have shown that

vigorous control of blood pressure and tight glycaemic control can reverse the microalbuminuria and slow the progression of frank proteinuria.

5. **B – Autonomic neuropathy**
Postural hypotension occurs as a result of autonomic neuropathy which, although it is extremely common in patients who have had diabetes for a number of years, does not often cause symptoms. Other manifestations include tachycardia, loss of sinus arrhythmia, gastroparesis, small-bowel bacterial overgrowth, denervation of the bladder and impotence.

6. DIABETIC EYE DISEASE

1. **A – Background retinopathy**
Diabetic retinopathy is a microvascular disease state with many similarities to diabetic nephropathy and, indeed, the two conditions often co-exist. Tight glycaemic control and blood-pressure control have been demonstrated both to delay the onset and to slow progression of retinopathy. In its earliest form, capillary weakening and destruction occurs, resulting in microaneurysm formation, blot haemorrhages and deposits of extravasated lipid, known as 'hard exudates'. If the macula is affected, the condition is known as 'diabetic maculopathy' and laser photocoagulation might be of value in preventing deterioration. If the macula is spared, these appearances are known as 'background retinopathy' and no ophthalmological treatment is indicated.

As the condition progresses, retinal ischaemia develops, resulting in retinal oedema, which is visible as hazy-margined pale areas known as 'cotton-wool spots'. Venous loops and beading also occur. This condition is known as 'pre-proliferative retinopathy', and warrants referral to an ophthalmologist. If the disease is allowed to progress further, proliferative retinopathy results, with new-vessel formation. These new vessels, which are usually concentrated around the optic disc and adjacent to the temporal vessels, are fragile and prone to causing vitreous haemorrhage. Panretinal laser photocoagulation halts or even reverses vascular proliferation by destroying ischaemic retina, thereby reducing the formation of factors promoting angiogenesis.

2. **J – Vitreous haemorrhage**
Vitreous haemorrhage, occurring as a result of proliferative retinopathy, can cause floaters or complete loss of vision. It can also occur in severe hypertension, following retinal tears, or as a result of neovascularisation secondary to retinal branch vein occlusion. The haemorrhage might be resorbed over a period of months, allowing some return of vision, but further haemorrhage or tractional retinal detachment can supervene.

3. **H – Proliferative retinopathy**
See answer to question 1.

4. **B – Central retinal artery occlusion**
Atherosclerosis with thrombosis or thromboembolism can affect the central retinal artery. Sudden visual loss results, which is almost always permanent and is followed by optic atrophy after a few weeks. Acutely, the retinal vessels become thread-like on fundoscopy. Retinal oedema causes the fundus to appear pale except at the macula where, because the retina is so thin, the red colour of the choroidal circulation is

visible. Other causes of central retinal artery occlusion include giant-cell arteritis and embolism from cardiac vegetations.

5. **C – Central retinal vein occlusion**
Central retinal vein occlusion occurs in diabetes mellitus, hypertension and systemic disease associated with a pro-thrombotic state, such as malignancy. Unlike central retinal artery occlusion, some improvement in vision sometimes occurs as the dramatic fundus signs resolve.

7. DRUG COMPLICATIONS IN PATIENTS WITH DIABETES

1. **A – Acarbose**
Acarbose is an intestinal α-glucosidase inhibitor that delays carbohydrate absorption, so reducing post-prandial hyperglycaemia. Its principal side-effects are intestinal, but it can rarely cause hepatic dysfunction.

2. **H – Propranolol**
Impending hypoglycaemia causes catecholamine release; awareness of the resulting symptoms is reduced by β-blockers, especially non-selective ones such as propranolol. In addition, β-blockers tend to cause a small deterioration in insulin resistance. When human insulin was first introduced, some users of animal-derived insulins found that their awareness of impending hypoglycaemia was reduced after conversion. Nowadays, the vast majority of patients with newly diagnosed diabetes mellitus are started on human insulin, with no such problems.

3. **D – Chlorpropamide**
Chlorpropamide is a member of the sulphonylurea group of drugs, which act by promoting endogenous insulin secretion and by increasing peripheral insulin sensitivity. The main side-effect of all sulphonylureas is hypoglycaemia, the risk of which increases with the half-life of the drug. Chlorpropamide is now seldom used because it has an unusually long half-life of 36 hours. In addition, chlorpropamide, uniquely among the sulphonylureas, causes an increase in ADH secretion and is also responsible for an unpleasant facial flushing after alcohol ingestion in a third of patients. The tendency to this adverse effect is inherited in an autosomal dominant fashion and is thought to be mediated by endorphins because it is blocked by naloxone.

4. **C – Bendroflumethiazide**
Thiazide diuretics cause an increase in serum glucose, lipids and uric acid. Fortunately, this effect is limited when low doses (eg bendroflumethiazide 2.5 mg once daily) are used but it is still advisable to avoid thiazides in patients with diabetes mellitus if possible. Unless contraindications are present, an ACE inhibitor is a good first choice for treating hypertension in the context of diabetes mellitus, especially if the patient has diabetic nephropathy.

5. **G – Metformin**
Metformin acts by promoting peripheral glucose uptake and reducing hepatic gluconeogenesis in the presence of endogenous insulin. Because it does not increase insulin secretion, it does not promote obesity and it does not cause hypoglycaemia.

Besides minor gastrointestinal side-effects, its main drawback is a propensity to cause lactic acidosis, especially in patients under stress (eg from infection, dehydration, myocardial infarction or surgery). The risk is greater in the presence of renal impairment. In these situations the drug is stopped and, if necessary, antidiabetic treatment is continued with insulin.

8. ADVERSE EFFECTS OF ENDOCRINE DRUGS

1.   C – Carbimazole
This woman has agranulocytosis, a rare complication of carbimazole treatment that renders the patient prone to overwhelming bacterial infection and sepsis. For this reason, patients prescribed carbimazole should be warned to seek medical attention if they develop symptoms or signs of infection, particularly a sore throat. A full blood count with white cell differential should always be performed, and the drug should be stopped if there is evidence of neutropenia.

2.   H – Octreotide
Octreotide is an analogue of somatostatin, the hypothalamus-derived inhibitor of growth hormone release. Its principal uses are in the symptomatic relief of acromegaly and gut peptide-releasing tumours and in down-regulation of pancreatic exocrine function after pancreatic surgery. Cholelithiasis is a well-recognised complication of long-term treatment with this drug.

3.   D – Chlorpropamide
Chlorpropamide enhances the action of vasopressin in the kidney, so promotes water retention. Symptomatic hyponatraemia is very rare but the side-effect is occasionally of clinical use in the management of partial cranial diabetes insipidus.

4.   E – Clomifene
Clomifene is an anti-oestrogen that is used in the treatment of anovulatory infertility. Ovarian hyperstimulation is a rare complication that presents with diffuse lower abdominal pain. Ascites, hydrothorax and venous and arterial thrombosis can all occur.

5.   A – Alendronate
Alendronate is a member of the bisphosphonate group of drugs and is used particularly in the treatment of postmenopausal osteoporosis. It can cause severe oesophagitis and oesophageal erosions and ulcers and patients are advised to swallow the tablets with a full glass of water and to remain standing or sit upright for half an hour afterwards.

9. LUMPS IN THE BREAST

1.   F – Fibrocystic change
Fibrocystic change is the most common disorder of the breast, estimates suggesting that at least 10% of women develop clinically apparent disease. The condition occurs most frequently between the ages of 20 and 40 and is rare before adolescence or after the menopause. A relative imbalance between oestrogen and progesterone during each

menstrual cycle is an important aetiological factor. The epithelium of the affected areas is hormonally sensitive, leading to fluctuation in size and tenderness according to the phase of the menstrual cycle.

2. **H – Invasive ductal carcinoma**
The main differential diagnosis of a stellate mass with microcalcification lies between an invasive carcinoma and a radial scar. The fact that this patient has enlarged ipsi-lateral axillary nodes suggests an invasive carcinoma with nodal metastases. Carcinoma of the breast comprises 20% of all cancers in women and is the commonest cause of death from malignancy in women aged between 35 and 55. Ductal carci-nomas constitute 75% of all invasive breast carcinomas, while lobular carcinomas comprise 10%; other types are rare.

3. **C – Duct ectasia**
Duct ectasia is a purely inflammatory condition with no relationship to malignancy. It usually involves the large subareolar ducts, which are dilated and filled with viscid white material. It can be difficult to distinguish duct ectasia from intraduct papilloma – both conditions present with nipple discharge that can be bloodstained and both are common in middle-aged women. In duct ectasia, however, cytological examination of the discharge shows macrophages and debris as the lesion is inflammatory; in intraduct papilloma, epithelial cells are seen because the lesion is a neoplasm. The pathogenesis of duct ectasia is unknown.

4. **E – Fibroadenoma**
Fibroadenoma is the commonest benign tumour of the breast and occurs most frequently in young women. Fibroadenomas arise from the breast lobule and are mixed tumours, containing both glandular epithelium and connective tissue stroma. Like areas of fibrocystic change, the epithelium of a fibroadenoma is hormonally responsive, so there can be a slight increase in size during the second half of the menstrual cycle. Unlike fibrocystic change, however, fibroadenomas are well circumscribed and solid with a lobulated appearance macroscopically. Fibroadenomas are not tethered to the surrounding breast tissue and this accounts for their mobility on palpation.

5. **A – Acute pyogenic mastitis**
Acute pyogenic mastitis is a painful inflammatory condition that usually occurs in the immediate post-partum period. *Staphylococcus aureus* is the most common causative organism and the usual portal of entry is a crack in the nipple. The infection tends to be confined to one segment of the breast, giving rise to localised swelling and erythema. If antibiotics are given without adequate drainage, a localised breast abscess will result.

10. GENERAL RASHES

1. **C – Erythema ab igne**
This patient has developed the classic reticular pattern of erythema ab igne. This is commonly seen in elderly patients or in those with cold intolerance who sit or lie too near to a heat source such as an electric fire or hot-water bottle. It has no pathological significance of its own.

2.   J – Rosacea

This woman has developed rosacea, an erythematous rash affecting the face, classically in the 'sign of the cross' (ie from the forehead down to the chin and horizontally across the cheeks). It can be preceded by a long history of flushing when stressed or hot and when drinking alcohol. Chronically, it can be associated with rhinophyma and telangiectasia. Treatment includes antibiotics and topical steroids.

3.   H – Necrobiosis lipoidica

Necrobiosis lipoidica is a relatively rare complication of diabetes mellitus and is thought to be due to small-vessel disease, although 50% of cases actually occur in pre- or non-diabetic patients. The condition causes partial necrosis of the dermal collagen and connective tissue and leads to a waxy, pigmented-looking lesion, often over the anterior shins. Although it is a self-limiting condition, the lesions are often slow to heal and might require intradermal steroids or even excision and skin grafting.

4.   G – Lupus vulgaris

This patient has pulmonary tuberculosis and has subsequently developed lupus vulgaris. This scaling, erythematous, plaque-like rash usually occurs through haematological spread from a primary lesion. Biopsy can demonstrate granulomatous infiltration associated with tubercles. Antituberculous therapy is required for 6–9 months.

5.   B – Dermatitis herpetiformis

Dermatitis herpetiformis can occur in isolation as in this case, or in association with coeliac disease. It can occur at any age, although the peak incidence is in the third to fourth decades. Many patients with isolated dermatitis herpetiformis have asymptomatic changes of the small bowel and gastrointestinal symptoms are rare. Both conditions share common HLA markers, abnormal IgA activity and both are associated with an increased risk of developing upper gastrointestinal malignancies. Treatment includes a gluten-free diet and dapsone.

11. BLISTERING RASHES

1.   I – Stevens–Johnson syndrome

This patient has developed Stevens–Johnson syndrome secondary to his chest infection. This is a 'malignant' form of erythema multiforme and can cause systemic upset. It involves the mucosal membranes and the eyes. The underlying cause needs to be treated but patients can require steroids and intravenous fluids.

2.   A – Dermatitis herpetiformis

This patient has coeliac disease with dermatitis herpetiformis, which can present as a blistering rash. Treatment includes a gluten-free diet and some patients require dapsone.

3.   D – Herpes zoster virus

This rash is dermatomal (approximately T10) and is due to herpes zoster, a reactivation of a previous varicella infection. Stress, illness and sunlight can all precipitate an infection. Early treatment with aciclovir is recommended to reduce the risk of post-herpetic neuralgia, which itself can cause great distress.

4.   **F – Pemphigoid**
Pemphigoi**d** is a bullous disorder affecting the **d**ermis (ie **d**eep lesions). The blisters are variable in size but are tense, and there will be a few de-roofed lesions. It rarely affects the mucous membranes and although self-limiting, patients often require steroid treatment for 1–2 years (with bone-sparing agents).

5.   **G – Pemphigus**
Pemphigu**S** produces **S**uperficial blisters based in the epidermis. The blisters are often deroofed and the underlying skin is thus denuded and tender. There may be lesions around the eyes, mucosal membranes and genitalia. Patients with pemphigus require high doses of steroids and immunosuppressants.

12. DERMATITIS

1.   **B – Atopic eczema**
Atopic eczema usually develops in the first 6 months of life but can present in later childhood. It will improve slowly over childhood and rarely occurs after early adolescence. Around 30–50% of patients have other atopic disorders, including asthma, hay fever, and food and medication allergies. Classically, it is intensely pruritic and affects the flexures and face. Chronically affected areas become dry and thickened, known as 'lichenification'.

2.   **G – Pityriasis alba**
Pityriasis alba is a low-grade eczematous rash that causes drying and subsequent skin shedding and depigmentation.

3.   **A – Asteatotic eczema**
Asteatotic eczema occurs commonly in the elderly and malnourished people when they are transferred into a warm environment such as a hospital ward. It occurs on exposed areas of skin and is exacerbated by irritants such as soap. Treatment includes weak topical steroid preparations and emollients.

4.   **C – Contact dermatitis**
This young man has developed a contact dermatitis. This is an allergic response to an environmental agent such as shampoo or other hair products. Common causative agents include cosmetics, nickel and chromium, rubber products and plants. Treatment includes stress reduction, avoidance of causative agents, and topical steroids. Rarely, immunosuppressant agents are required.

5.   **F – Nummular dermatitis**
Nummular eczema is characterised by symmetrical round lesions or patches of eczema. These can be vesicular and extremely pruritic. This condition can occur as an allergic response to insect bites or to nickel and chromium products.

13. PRURITUS

1. I – Scabies
This man has developed scabies, characterised by intense pruritus and the 'burrows' between the fingers. Affected individuals become sensitised to the female mite of *Sarcoptes scabiei* and develop tracts along which the mite has burrowed. A more 'malignant' form can occur in immunocompromised patients and this is known as 'Norwegian scabies'.

2. G – Lymphoma
This woman has developed pruritus secondary to her lymphoma. Systemic features such as weight loss and night sweats are called 'B'-symptoms. They can occur at any stage of the disease but are more likely in advanced stages.

3. H – Psoriasis
This woman has all the classic features of a psoriatic rash. In any chronic skin condition, pruritus is caused by drying of the skin and can be avoided with good control, emollients and avoidance of irritants such as soap.

4. E – Iron deficiency
This man has features suggestive of a gastric carcinoma with secondary iron deficiency. Iron deficiency is a relatively common cause of pruritus in the elderly and should initially be treated with oral iron preparations. Investigations include upper and lower gastrointestinal endoscopy, barium studies or abdominal CT.

5. J – Uraemia
This man has developed uraemia secondary to his ACE-inhibitor treatment, which has caused renal failure. Other signs of uraemia include uraemic frost on the skin, confusion, seizures, depressed level of consciousness, pericarditis and hiccups.

14. CHANGE IN PIGMENTATION

1. D – Ectopic ACTH secretion
This patient has an ectopic ACTH-producing bronchial (probably small-cell) carcinoma. The ectopic ACTH causes a Cushing's syndrome marked principally by oedema, hyperpigmentation and hypokalaemia. The patient often complains of severe lethargy and weakness because of the profound hypokalaemia and proximal myopathy.

2. I – Pityriasis versicolor
Pityriasis versicolor is a fungal rash caused by *Malassezia furfur*, a parasitic form of the saprophytic yeast *Pityrosporum orbiculare*. The yeast produces a melanocyte inhibitor and so the rash is often noticed when pale-skinned patients are exposed to sunlight. The lesions are scaling, macular and confluent and might even be hyperpigmented.

3. J – Vitiligo
This patient has vitiligo, which is thought to be an autoimmune phenomenon associated with melanocyte destruction. The areas of hypopigmentation are usually well demarcated and symmetrical. The phenomenon is associated with other autoimmune disorders, such as pernicious anaemia and thyroid disease, as well as with diabetes

mellitus. It is a common incidental finding and should alert the examiner to the possibilities of these associations.

4. **B – Addison's disease**
This patient has developed Addison's disease, as evidenced by the low blood sugar, hypotension and hyperpigmentation of the skin creases and scar. The hyperpigmentation is often marked at sites of trauma (eg below waistbands or bra straps), and is also commonly seen in the buccal mucosa.

5. **A – Acanthosis nigricans**
This patient has acanthosis nigricans, which can be associated with underlying malignancy, classically gastric carcinoma. In younger patients it can be associated with obesity, insulin-resistant states, and endocrine disorders such as acromegaly and polycystic ovary syndrome.

15. NAIL DISORDERS

1. **A, I – Clubbing and splinter haemorrhages**
This patient has developed infective endocarditis, as evidenced by the low-grade fever, the Osler's nodes, the new systolic murmur and the evidence of cardiac failure. The expected nail changes are splinter haemorrhages, which occur at the nail fold, and clubbing, although this takes many months to develop.

2. **E – Onycholysis**
This patient has developed thyrotoxicosis with associated onycholysis or splitting of the distal nail. This condition can also occur in psoriasis and after trauma to the nail.

3. **A, C – Clubbing and leuconychia**
This gentleman has signs consistent with chronic alcoholic liver disease. Cirrhosis is associated with hypoalbuminaemia, causing leuconychia or white nails, and clubbing.

4. **D – Onychogryphosis**
Onychogryphosis is a due to neglect, trauma or, rarely, ischaemia. It represents an overgrowth and thickening, leading to disfigurement of the nails. It is commonly seen in disabled elderly people who are unable to look after their nails: this is simply remedied by regular visits to the chiropodist.

5. **A – Clubbing**
This patient has developed bronchiectasis, which is associated with clubbing of the nails.

16. ERYTHEMA NODOSUM

Erythema nodosum is a painful, erythematous, tender rash that principally occurs over the anterior shins. Lesions are often ill-defined and can coalesce. It can also occur over the forearms and, more rarely, truncal areas.

1. **H – Sarcoidosis**
    This man has developed sarcoidosis, as evidenced by the bilateral hilar lymphadenopathy and the raised serum calcium. Although bilateral hilar lymphadenopathy can occur in lymphoma or tuberculosis these are unlikely with the presenting symptoms, raised serum calcium and raised ACE.

2. **J – Tuberculosis**
    This gentleman has developed pulmonary tuberculosis. Sarcoid and tuberculosis are the commonest causes of erythema nodosum in the UK.

3. **D – Hodgkin's disease**
    This young woman has developed Hodgkin's lymphoma. Epstein–Barr virus infection has a well-recognised association with Burkitt's lymphoma but there also seems to be a causal link in up to 30% of patients with Hodgkin's disease. The normocytic anaemia, raised ESR and peripheral lymphocytosis are characteristic of the early stages of the disease.

4. **B – Epstein–Barr virus**
    This young woman has developed glandular fever, caused by the Epstein–Barr virus. The monospot test is the detection of atypical mononuclear cells in a peripheral blood film. Later confirmation can be obtained by a positive Paul–Bunnell test, which demonstrates the presence of the IgM associated with the infection.

5. **I – *Streptococcus***
    This elderly man has developed a classic lobar pneumonia secondary to a streptococcal infection. *Streptococcus* is the commonest cause of pneumonia in the UK and is still extremely virulent. Without early treatment it can be life-threatening, particularly in the elderly. Patients requiring admission to hospital with pneumonia should always be covered for streptococcal infection with appropriate antibiotics (eg penicillin, cephalosporins or clarithromycin).

17. ERYTHEMA MULTIFORME

Erythema multiforme is characterised by erythematous 'target' lesions, which are annular and blistering. It is principally a peripheral rash which can become more generalised. A severe form of the rash, Stevens–Johnson syndrome, causes a bullous-type eruption associated with fever, anorexia and oral, genital and ophthalmic lesions. Around 50% of cases are idiopathic, with the commonest identifiable cause being herpes simplex virus (HSV) infection and other infections. Most drugs and infectious agents are thought to be able to cause erythema multiforme, usually after a latent period of 1–2 weeks. The other listed causes are relatively uncommon.

1. **G – *Streptococcus***
    This young boy has developed streptococcal meningitis with an associated erythema multiforme. Severe streptococcal meningitis can cause a purpuric rash classically seen in meningococcal disease. The high CSF protein concentration and low glucose concentration are characteristic of a bacterial meningitis.

2. **D –** *Mycoplasma*
    This patient presents clinical features, along with the hyponatraemia, deranged LFTs and the radiographic features, that are highly suggestive of an atypical pneumonia, in this case a *Mycoplasma* pneumonia.

3. **J – Ulcerative colitis**
    This patient has inflammatory bowel disease, which is occasionally associated with erythema multiforme. Other dermatological lesions associated with inflammatory bowel disease are erythema nodosum, pyoderma gangrenosum and vasculitic changes.

4. **H – SLE**
    This patient has SLE, which can cause erythema multiforme. Other dermatological lesions associated with this condition include vasculitis, discoid lupus, a photosensitivity rash, livedo reticularis, alopecia and Raynaud's phenomenon.

5. **B – Herpes simplex virus**
    This patient has a healing herpes simplex lesion on the upper lip. HSV type 1 is the commonest identifiable cause of erythema multiforme and can be responsible for recurrent outbreaks of the condition. Early treatment with aciclovir is recommended.

18. PYODERMA GANGRENOSUM

Pyoderma gangrenosum is a necrotising, ulcerating lesion which initially starts as papular and pustular areas that rapidly coalesce and enlarge to form the typical necrotic ulcer. More rarely, it starts as a bullous eruption. As with erythema multiforme, 50% of cases are idiopathic, and there is no known link between the other causes.

1. **J – Wegener's granulomatosis**
    This patient has Wegener's granulomatosis. Pyoderma is commonly linked to vasculitic conditions and an autoantibody screen should be sent off whenever investigating patients with this condition.

2. **E – Myelofibrosis**
    This woman has developed myelofibrosis. The absence of the Philadelphia chromosome and the unsuccessful bone marrow aspiration help to differentiate it from chronic myeloid leukaemia, which can present in a similar manner.

3. **I – Waldenström's macroglobulinaemia**
    Patients with Waldenström's macroglobulinaemia present with symptoms secondary to their bone marrow failure (ie anaemia, infections, bruising and bleeding). It can be differentiated from multiple myeloma by the absence of lytic bone lesions, normocalcaemia, and the characteristic presence of an IgM paraproteinaemia. The disease has a much more benign course than myeloma and patients might only require supportive blood transfusions in the early stages.

4. **B – Ankylosing spondylitis**
    This patient has ankylosing spondylitis, a seronegative arthropathy that characteristically affects young men. Treatment should include physiotherapy and daily back exercises,

which are extremely important. NSAIDs are the other mainstay of therapy; immunosuppressants do not have a useful role.

5. **H – Ulcerative colitis**

    This patient has ulcerative colitis, as evidenced by the history and histology report, which differentiates it from Crohn's disease. Pyoderma can precede gastrointestinal symptoms but can occur at any stage of the disease. It occurs in about 3% of patients with ulcerative colitis and is unrelated to disease activity.

ANSWERS TO CHAPTER – PAEDIATRICS 5

1. INTERVENTIONS FOR ABNORMAL HEART RHYTHM

There are only a few treatment options for dysrhythmias in children at this level – vagal manoeuvres, adenosine, adrenaline (epinephrine), shocks and cardiopulmonary resuscitation (CPR). Agents such as amiodarone and other anti-arrhythmics are used in consultation with a paediatric cardiologist. Atropine can speed up the heart, but bradycardia is usually caused by hypoxia in children.

1. **I – No intervention from this list**
This question is assessing whether you know the age-appropriate values for vital signs. If you know these (newborn heart rate 110–160 bpm, respiratory rate <40 breaths/minute), you will spot the low heart rate. Here it appears that the infant is well apart from the low heart rate. This cannot be hypoxia as the oxygen saturation is 98%. Atropine could be given, but there would be no point, and the correct approach would be to wait and see what happens. If the situation does not change, an electrocardiogram (ECG) might show there is heart block.

2. **F – Bag-valve-mask ventilation**
This question is assessing whether you know the neonatal resuscitation protocol. After drying, the infant should be oxygenated, and as he is apnoeic, this will be by bag-valve-mask ventilation at first. The pallor is due to catecholamine-driven vasoconstriction. Cardiac massage should then be started, followed by intubation and adrenaline (epinephrine) via the endotracheal tube or an umbilical venous line.

3. **I – No intervention from this list**
This patient is shocked, so has a sinus tachycardia. The most appropriate management is to give fluid boluses. Diabetic ketoacidosis can derange electrolytes, with an elevated potassium at presentation and a low potassium after insulin is started, and it is possible that an electrolyte disturbance has caused the tachycardia. If the tachycardia does not begin to settle with fluid boluses, then an ECG might help exclude a dysrhythmia.

4. **D – Asynchronous shock**
Tachycardia in children is either sinus (ie secondary to another cause), or primary. The commonest cause is supraventricular tachycardia, which can occur in otherwise normal hearts, or it could be ventricular tachycardia, which is almost always found with either a myocardial infection or following an operation. Here there is pulseless ventricular tachycardia, which is treated in the same way as ventricular fibrillation, with asynchronous shocks and then intravenous adrenaline.

5. **A – Intravenous adenosine**
This patient is most likely to have a supraventricular tachycardia, and the ECG would be expected to show a narrow-complex tachycardia. This can be terminated with vagal manoeuvres, such as placing the infants head (briefly) in a bucket of cold water, but, failing this, adenosine is useful both to diagnose the problem and terminate the tachycardia. Adenosine is metabolised rapidly and will arrest the dysrhythmia at least for a few seconds if it is not ventricular in origin.

2. CAUSES OF HYPERTENSION

Hypertension in children is almost always secondary to another cause – and there are only seven causes to choose from. Two of the seven restrict blood flow to the kidney and so there is a compensatory overactivity in the renin–angiotensin system – these are coarctation of the aorta and renal artery stenosis. Four pathological causes lead to hypertension because of hormonal disorders – phaeochromocytomas, neuroblastomas, congenital adrenal hyperplasia and, of course, steroid and other drug administration. Primary kidney disease can also lead to hypertension.

1. **F – Iatrogenic**
Corticosteroids form an important part of the treatment of haematological and brain tumours. However this part of the question also contains a lot of other clinical data that suggest that there could be other disease present. On closer inspection, the features are all consistent with leukaemia. The murmur is a typical 'innocent' murmur, and is probably caused by the anaemia. It could be possible that the child has infective endocarditis, giving rise to the murmur, and the petechial rash might be microemboli, but this would not cause hypertension and is exceedingly unlikely (even for an EMQ!).

2. **A – Coarctation of the aorta**
Only two murmurs radiate to the back – that of a patent ductus arteriosus and that of coarctation of the aorta. A murmur will radiate in the direction that the blood is flowing in at the site of turbulence. A patent ductus gives a wide pulse pressure (blood flows in diastole into the low-pressure pulmonary circuit, so the diastolic blood pressure is low). One of the causes of short stature in a girl is Turner's syndrome (XO), which is associated with left-sided heart defects – aortic stenosis and coarctation.

3. **E – Haemolytic-uraemic syndrome**
This is a description of haemolytic-uraemic syndrome (HUS), an important cause of acute renal failure in children. This is a toxin-mediated disease, and *Escherichia coli* O157 is the most common source. It is characterised by microangiopathic haemolytic anaemia, uraemia and thrombocytopenia.

4. **B – Congenital adrenal hyperplasia**
Most children with delayed puberty do not have a disorder but children presented in exams are more likely to have a range of other conditions – pituitary or brain tumours or hormone production or insensitivity disorders. Congenital adrenal hyperplasia comprises a group of conditions in which there is a defect in the production of steroid hormones (cortisol, sex steroids, aldosterone) in the adrenal cortex. Feedback mechanisms to the hypothalamus and pituitary increase secretion of ACTH, which in turn attempts to increase production of these hormones, and also leads to hypertrophy of the adrenal cortex. Clinical manifestations include (depending on the defect) ambiguous genitalia, salt-wasting with shock, and hypertension.

5. **G – Neuroblastoma**
A painless abdominal mass in a child is a Wilms' tumour, a neuroblastoma, an enlarged polycystic kidney, or perhaps a lymphoma. Neuroblastomas often arise in the adrenal gland and can press directly onto the kidney causing hypertension. They can also secrete catecholamine-like hormones that are vasoactive.

3. CHOICE OF ANTIBIOTIC

Paediatricians commonly treat children with infections, but the range of organisms encountered is quite small. Antibiotic policies have now been simplified and rationalised in most hospitals to cover the expected organisms. Seriously ill children are given intravenous ceftriaxone or cefotaxime, and neonates are treated with penicillin and gentamicin. Children with urinary tract infections are given trimethoprim or, if they are ill, ceftriaxone. Other situations are outlined below.

1. **C – Intravenous co-amoxiclav (Augmentin®)**
Community-acquired chest infection is often viral. If bacterial, it is usually caused by *Streptococcus pneumoniae* (pneumococcus) but is occasionally caused by unencapsulated *Haemophilus influenzae*. In children aged over 5 years, *Mycoplasma* becomes more important. Chest infection is best treated with amoxicillin, with the addition of azithromycin or a similar agent in over-5s. The child in the question will have an impaired cough and is clearly pretty sick. This makes infection with *Staphylococcus aureus* more likely, which is treated with co-amoxiclav. This is effective against pneumococci and most community-acquired staphylococci, as well as being active against anaerobic organisms. *Mycoplasma* is not thought to give rise to severe infections.

2. **J – Oral vancomycin**
Post-antibiotic diarrhoea is very common, caused by changes in gut bacterial flora. The severity of her symptoms and the identification of *Clostridium difficile* toxin suggests that she has pseudomembranous colitis. This is treated with oral metronidazole or oral vancomycin. Vancomycin is not absorbed from the gut.

3. **D – Intravenous vancomycin**
A coagulase-negative staphylococcus is usually *Staphylococcus epidermidis,* an organism of low infectivity found on the skin. It is usually resistant to penicillins and co-amixiclav. Only patients with impaired immunity will contract an invasive infection, but indwelling lines can become colonised. Sometimes, treatment with intravenous vancomycin does not clear the infection and the line must be removed.

4. **A – Intraveous benzylpenicillin and gentamicin**
Group B *Streptococcus*, *Listeria* and Gram-negative organisms are responsible for almost all early neonatal infections. These can be treated with benzylpenicillin and gentamicin together. Any suspicion of a neonatal infection should prompt a comprehensive infection screen and the baby should always receive these antibiotics, as the signs are often subtle.

5. **E – No intervention from this list**
Most upper respiratory tract infections are viral. Children who are more unwell, who have pus on their tonsils, or who have only one inflamed tympanic membrane are more likely to have a bacterial cause, but there is little evidence for this, or for using antibiotics in this setting. An exception might be if there was impaired immunity, where a broad-spectrum agent should be used, or if the throat alone was very inflamed, in which case penicillin V should be used after a swab has been taken.

4. CAUSES OF LYMPHADENOPATHY

Lymphadenopathy is either generalised or local, tender or non-tender. Lymphadenopathey caused by a local problem is, predictably, found in the area of lymphatic drainage, and haematological or systemic disorders produce generalised lymphadenopathy. Tender nodes result from inflammation, usually infection. Non-tender nodes are suggestive of infiltration, probably malignant.

1. H – Reaction to local infection
Seborrheic dermatitis (cradle cap) can become very inflamed and even infected, causing local lymphadenopathy.

2. C – Cat scratch disease
Cat scratch disease is rarely seen in those aged over 20 years. A lick or bite from a cat leads to local infection with *Bartonella henselae*. A small papule or red pustule is seen at the site of bacterial entry. Two weeks later, nearby lymph nodes become inflamed and swell. Only symptomatic treatment is needed in most cases.

3. D – Epstein–Barr viral infection
Many infections cause widespread lymphadenopathy – HIV, rubella, CMV and, most commonly, EBV. Lymphadenopathy and pharyngitis are the most common symptoms with EBV infection, but hepato- or splenomegaly, a rash and jaundice can also occur.

4. E – HIV infection
Coming from Uganda in an examination suggests HIV or tuberculosis, although of course most children coming from Africa are healthy. Parasite infections or malaria will also be important examination topics in such patients. HIV can present in a variety of ways in childhood – *Pneumocystis carinii* pneumonia (PCP) as a neonate or infant, growth faltering, malabsorption, encephalopathy, lymphadenopathy or parotitis.

5. A – Acute lymphoblastic leukaemia
Petechial rash is caused by thrombocytopenia (due to leukaemia or idiopathic thrombocytopenic purpura) or vasculitis (due to meningococcal infection or Henoch–Schönlein purpura). Recurrent respiratory infections suggest asthma, cystic fibrosis or an immune deficiency.

5. INFECTING ORGANISMS

Infecting organisms in neonates were discussed in theme 3. In older children, invasive infection is typically caused one of by just three organisms – *Neisseria meningitidis*, *Streptococcus pneumoniae* or *Haemophilus influenzae* type B (HIB). HIB tends to affect under-5s and pneumococcus affects older children, although the introduction of HIB immunisation has dramatically reduced the incidence of HIB infection. These three organisms can cause septicaemia or meningitis in previously healthy children.

1. **G –** *Staphylococcus aureus*
   Staphylococcus aureus and *Streptococcus pyogenes* (group A streptococcus) cause most skin infections. Both can cause cellulitis, and staphylococci can also cause abscesses. Eczema can become infected with *S. aureus* and can also be exacerbated by chickenpox.

2. **H –** *Staphylococcus epidermidis* (**coagulase-negative staphylococcus**)
   Bacterial infections usually make children very ill. Children on chemotherapy are at high risk of invasive bacterial infection with a wide range of organisms of varying pathogenicity. The most common infection in children with indwelling catheters is with *S. epidermidis*. This can become a systemic infection but, if confined to the line itself, causes fever and inflammation around the line.

3. **F –** *Salmonella enteritidis*
   Of the organisms in the list, only *Eshcerichia coli* and *Salmonella* are likely to cause gastrointestinal infection, with *Salmonella* the more common in non-travellers. The severity also suggests that this is a *Salmonella* infection. This organism can cause bloody diarrhoea.

4. **I –** *Streptococcus pneumoniae* (**pneumococcus**)
   Fever with a change in consciousness is caused by meningitis, encephalitis or a cerebral abscess. Cerebral abscess must be excluded in a child like this with a CT scan, but it is relatively unlikely. Encephalitis is caused by viruses, particularly herpes simplex virus. Meningitis is usually bacterial, and caused by *Neisseria meningitidis*, *Streptococcus pneumoniae* or *Haemophilus influenzae* type B. The patient's age and the lack of a rash make pneumococcus the most likely organism here.

5. **I –** *Streptococcus pneumoniae* (**pneumococcus**)
   Pneumococcus and unencapsulated *Haemophilus* (ie not HIB) are the most likely bacterial causes of chest infection in children. *Mycoplasma* is more likely to cause widespread diffuse changes in the radiograph, rather than lobar changes seen here.

6. CAUSES OF APNOEA

Apnoea is a common presentation for a large and diverse range of conditions affecting neonates and young infants. Other symptoms, signs and investigations are used to distinguish between the different infections and other causes.

1. **F – Meningitis**
   Premature babies have a very poor immune system. Invasive bacterial infection is common but the signs are subtle. Signs such as apnoeas, low or high temperature, high or low glucose, change in respiratory function, feed intolerance or even how the infant is handling can all indicate infection. In reality, this infant might also have pneumonia, or indeed septicaemia instead of meningitis because these conditions will present similarly. Apnoea of prematurity or reflux would not make the baby sleepy. Apnoea of prematurity is very common, but a diagnosis of exclusion, and no other symptoms would be expected.

2. **E – Gastro-oesophageal reflux disease**
Symptoms related to feeds are often caused by reflux – these can include vomiting, coughing, arching of the back and apnoeas. Again, apnoea of prematurity could be a possible cause.

3. **D – Bronchiolitis**
In normal term infants, apnoeas can be caused by serious infections such as meningitis, but more often bronchiolitis, reflux or pertussis will be the cause. Hyperexpansion of the lungs is caused by small-airways disease, and this is most likely to be bronchiolitis or asthma. The age of the infant makes asthma impossible.

4. **H – Pertussis**
Pertussis is a serious infection in the very young, and can cause severe hypoxia and cerebral haemorrhages. In older children it can simply present as a persistent cough.

5. **J – Seizure**
Seizures in neonates are difficult to spot. This is partly because the lack of myelination means that typical tonic-clonic fits do not occur. Instead, convulsions can manifest as apnoeas, lip-smacking, cycling or repetitive movements. In this child, meningitis might also have led to the fetal distress that was identified before delivery and to the seizures, so this would need to be excluded.

7. USING INVESTIGATIONS

Paediatricians like to think that they are particularly judicious over their use of invasive investigations and ionising radiation. Each test needs to be justified in terms of a potential change in management and benefit to the child.

1. **A or F – CT scan of the brain or MRI scan of the brain**
The history is strongly suggestive of raised intracranial pressure. Acute central nervous system (CNS) changes are due to bleeds, acute hydrocephalus or infection. Subacute changes are more likely due to an intracranial tumour. CT scanning is particularly useful for looking at blood in the CSF, MRI scanning for differences in texture of tissue in the head. MRI is probably the best test for investigating subacute neurological changes, and CT for sudden changes. CT scans are easier to obtain. A lumbar puncture should not be attempted because of the risk of coning.

2. **I – Ultrasound of the brain**
At this age, a rapidly enlarging head is due to hydrocephalus, secondary to infection or blood in the CSF. Congenital anomalies in the drainage system can also cause hydrocephalus, but this will present antenatally or will have been identified at birth. As the sutures are not closed, an increase in the amount of CSF will directly expand the head without an increase in intracranial pressure. Ultrasound is excellent for differentiating between tissue and fluid, the essence of diagnosis of hydrocephalus. Unfortunately, it does not 'see' well through bone. However, the open anterior fontanelle will be open in this infant (this remains open up to 9 months).

3. **G – Paired urine/blood osmolality**

Respiratory illnesses, intracranial pathology and surgery all have the potential to lead to inappropriate ADH secretion. ADH promotes retention of water in the kidneys and can lead to hyponatraemia on 'standard' intravenous fluid regimens. Symptomatic hyponatraemia should be treated by infusion of 3% saline initially and then fluid restriction. It is diagnosed by comparing the serum and urine osmolalities – with inappropriate ADH, the urine is concentrated despite a hypotonic serum (<270 mOsmol/l).

4. **A – CT scan of the brain**

Drowsiness without shock, metabolic disturbance or drugs suggests intracranial pathology. In this setting, acute bleeding is most likely, especially as the child is becoming increasingly drowsy. A CT head scan is needed to determine if the child needs neurosurgery. Fundoscopy might reveal papilloedema (associated with raised intracranial pressure), but changes can take some hours to develop, and this would not help to diagnose the problem. Similarly, a skull radiograph will only show that there has been a fracture and will not explain a reduced Glasgow Coma Scale (GCS) or whether this has led to raised intracranial pressure.

5. **A – CT scan of the brain**

A febrile convulsion can only be diagnosed if other causes have been ruled out. This can be done clinically in most cases, as children with meningitis, encephalitis, an abscess or an underlying brain disorder are not normal before and after the seizure. So, if a child is outside the typical age range (6 months to 3 years), has a prolonged or focal convulsion, and is not neurologically normal before and after the fit, or is not developing normally, further investigations and antibiotics are indicated. A CT is the best way of looking for an abscess. A lumbar puncture would be useful, but this can be dangerous in an acutely drowsy child.

8. CAUSES OF ABDOMINAL DISTENSION

Abdominal distension in children is unlikely to be caused by fetus, but fluid, intestinal distension and masses are all possible. The causes are fairly distinct from those causing distension in adults.

1. **J – Wilms' tumour**

An abdominal mass in a child is most likely to be a Wilms' tumour, a neuroblastoma, polycystic kidneys or perhaps a lymphoma. Splenomegaly should be easy to distinguish from another mass. Appendicitis can lead to the development of a mass, but this would be accompanied by signs of local inflammation.

2. **G – Splenomegaly**

This description of the mass is typical of an enlarged spleen. Chronic splenomegaly is found in storage disorders, thalassaemia and haematological malignancies. Acute splenic enlargement can occur in a sequestration syndrome in sickle-cell disease.

3. **A – Appendicitis**

Many presentations in children are non-specific. Initially, this child might have had mesenteric adenitis, appendicitis, abdominal migraine or even a pneumonia, which often gives rise to referred pain in the abdomen. With the development of guarding and rigidity, however, there must be peritoneal inflammation. Absent bowel sounds will only occur if there is peritonitis, severe electrolyte disturbance or systemic infection.

4. D – Hirshprung's disease
Intestinal obstruction only causes distension if the blockage is sufficiently low, and the lower it is, the more distension is possible. This means that history and examination will enable you to distinguish between pyloric stenosis, duodenal atresia, other gut atresias and Hirschprung's disease, in which a lack of innervation of the myenteric plexus leads to constriction of the gut, preventing forward passage of stool. As the innervation process starts proximally and ends in the rectum, children who are mildly affected will have disease involving only a small part of the sigmoid colon; in severe disease, the entire colon is affected.

5. F – Nephrotic syndrome
Non-tender, generalised abdominal swelling is usually due to gaseous distension or to fluid. Ascites is typically caused by nephrotic syndrome, where leakage of albumin into the urine occurs at the glomerulus, leading to peripheral oedema and ascites.

9. INVESTIGATION OF RESPIRATORY DISTRESS

To work out which investigation is 'most useful in the management' requires the candidate to work out first what the diagnosis is, or so one would have thought. However, many options can be discounted immediately. For instance, the FEV_1 is a lung function test that a child aged under 5 years will not be able to perform. Similarly, the peak flow will not be possible in this age group (and it would only be of value after basic tests such as chest radiography). Other tests can only be used to make a specific diagnosis – the sweat test or pH probe for instance.

1. A – Bronchoscopy
Abrupt onset of respiratory symptoms suggests either a pneumothorax, reflux with aspiration, or an inhaled foreign body. Pneumothorax is very unusual except in asthmatics or after trauma. Reflux with aspiration only occurs in the very young, or those with abnormal neurology. An inhaled foreign body is most common in boys in their second year and will cause asymmetrical signs. Although inspiratory-expiratory chest radiographs can be useful diagnostically, this diagnosis can only be excluded by bronchoscopy.

2. F – Noctural oxygen saturation recording
Many children snore at night, and some might also have narrowing of the airways or enlarged tonsils as a cause. It is important to establish how severe the symptoms really are before embarking on further investigations or an operation. A sleep study to determine the amount of desaturated time can be used for this. The more sophisticated polysomnography simultaneously records saturation, heart rate, electroencephalogram, electromyogram and respiratory movements. It has become the definitive test for sleep apnoea.

3. G – None of the investigations listed
The main problem in this scenario is deciding whether the child needs a chest radiograph or not (remembering that the peak flow is not possible in such a young patient). The radiation dose of a chest radiograph is small, but the test must still be justified. All

asthmatics should have one at initial diagnosis to help exclude other causes of wheeze, such as infection or congenital lung malformations. Thereafter, asthmatic children do not need re-irradiation unless they have an atypical attack (asymmetric or unusual signs, particularly if severe or not improving on treatment).

4.   **J – Sweat test**
A child with recurrent chest infections is most likely to have cystic fibrosis, reflux with aspiration, an immunoglobulin deficiency or a lung malformation. Cystic fibrosis is also suggested by the poor weight gain. Of the choices available, a pH probe would not be totally wrong, but a barium swallow is a poor test to identify reflux. A sweat test is the most likely to find a diagnosis.

5.   **G – None of the investigations listed**
Congenital inspiratory stridor is usually due to largygeal floppiness or malacia of trachea. If stridor presents later it is most likely to be laryngotracheobronchitis (croup), but bacterial tracheitis and even epiglottitis are possible. In well children with mild symptoms, no intervention is needed; nebulised steroids are used in more severe cases. A nasopharyngeal aspirate might identify the causative virus.

10. CAUSES OF GROWTH FALTERING

Growth faltering used to be called 'failure to thrive' – weight gain or length gain below the expected. Normal growth requires adequate feeding and appetite, swallowing, intestinal function, normal digestion and metabolism, and no excessive energy demands. Control of growth is mediated by a number of hormones, each active at different ages.

1.   **A – Coeliac disease**
Weight faltering alone is not due to an endocrine disorder, rather inadequate energy supply or excessive needs. Here there is a strong suggestion that there is an intestinal cause. Of the possibilities available, congenital lactase deficiency and cystic fibrosis would have caused a problem earlier in life. Crohn's disease can occur at 13 months, but coeliac disease is much more common because it develops with the introduction of gluten into the diet during the first year.

2.   **C – Congestive cardiac failure**
Afro-Caribbeans have a very low incidence of cystic fibrosis. Hepatomegaly can be caused by liver disease, infiltration, haematological disorders or cardiac failure. The liver can also be pushed down by lung hyperexpansion. The clinical features in this child are those of congestive cardiac failure. The poor feeding occurs because the baby is too short of breath to be able to suck. Cystic fibrosis could also lead to these signs and symptoms, but this is less likely.

3.   **G – Growth hormone deficiency**
Height faltering more than weight faltering suggests a hormonal disorder. Thyroxine is the most important hormone for growth in children under 2 years, and growth hormone from then until puberty, when sex hormones become more important.

4. **I – Hypothyroidism**

Thyroid hormones are vital for the normal development of many tissues, and congenital hypothyroidism leads to poor brain growth and severe developmental delay.

5. **H – HIV infection**

This child has an infectious disorder in addition to poor weight gain. Cystic fibrosis is possible, but very unlikely with his racial origin. He might also have an immunoglobulin deficiency, but it is far more likely that he has HIV.

11. FLUID MANAGEMENT OF DIARRHOEA

Intravenous fluid used inappropriately can be dangerous. Remember that 0.9% NaCl is isotonic, but 0.45% NaCl / 5% dextrose, while near-isotonic at administration behaves as hypotonic fluid as soon as the dextrose is metabolised. During the dehydration of a child, initially the body restricts its own losses in urine and saliva. Once the child is over about 3% dehydrated, fluid moves out of cells to replace losses and restore circulating volume, and these shifts can be seen as a sunken fontanelle, sunken eyes and reduced tissue turgor. Once a child is over 10% dehydrated, such compensations can no longer maintain the circulating volume and shock develops, with poor perfusion, tachycardia and hypotension. Fluid boluses should be used to correct lack of circulating volume, but slower rehydration is more appropriate for cellular dehydration. It is almost always safer and more effective to start this as oral rehydration with Dioralyte® or oral rehydration solution (ORS) rather than intravenously. Sometimes vomiting is so severe that this in not effective and intravenous fluid is needed. Hypernatraemic dehydration means that all of the body's cells are hypertonic too, and rapid rehydration with a hypotonic solution has the potential to cause cerebral oedema.

1. **B – Dioralyte®**

This child is between 3% and 10% dehydrated. She needs rehydration, and the oral route should be tried first. If she is not improving because of her vomiting, intravenous rehydration with 0.9% NaCL over 24 hours can be used.

2. **B – Dioralyte®**

This child is very similar, but has hypernatraemic dehydration. A slower approach is needed, both to the oral rehydration and the intravenous rehydration if this is needed.

3. **B – Dioralyte®**

Despite the large number of stools, we are not told about any features of cellular dehydration and she is cardiovascularly stable. As she is not vomiting, oral rehydration is most appropriate. Milk feeding can be problematic during and after gastroenteritis because viral infection sometimes causes a temporary lactase deficiency, so that milk triggers an osmotic diarrhoea.

4. **D – Normal diet**

This child has no signs of any fluid or electrolyte disturbance.

5. **E – 0.9% NaCl Bolus over 20 minutes**

This child is shocked. The first priority is to restore the circulating volume with isotonic fluid – 0.9% saline or Hartmann's solution would be appropriate. Colloid would also restore the volume, but the child has a primary fluid and electrolyte disorder, so crystalloid is a better choice. After this, a choice between intravenous and oral rehydration can be made.

12. CAUSES OF ABNORMAL CARDIAC AUSCULTATION FINDINGS

Auscultation findings should only be interpreted along with other clinical features. That said, there are some useful guides that can be applied to children with murmurs. If loudest below the nipple line, the commonest murmurs are innocent (systolic only) or due to ventricular septal defects (VSDs) (pansystolic). Mitral regurgitation is rare in children, but will also cause a pansystolic murmur.

Above the nipple line, most murmurs are systolic as they come from the outflow tracts, where flow occurs in systole only. Aortic stenosis radiates to the neck, but pulmonary stenosis is hard to separate from a flow murmur. Coarctation gives rise to a murmur higher up, near the left clavicle, and this can radiate to the back. This is similar to a ductal murmur, but the ductal murmur can last longer, even through diastole. The blood pressure and distal pulses are completely different, with low-volume or delayed femoral pulses with hypertension in coarctation, and a bounding pulse with a wide pulse pressure with a patent ductus arteriosus (PDA).

1. **H – Pericardial rub**
    A scratchy noise ('like a mouse in the chest') in time with the cardiac cycle is a pericardial friction rub. Uraemia, tuberculosis and viral infections can lead to pericarditis but here it is caused by post-surgical inflammation.

2. **G – Patent ductus arteriosus**
    This murmur could also be caused by coarctation, although the question specifically avoids commenting on the femoral pulses or right-arm blood pressure, which would be abnormal in coarctiation.

3. **D – Coarctation of the aorta**
    This child appears to have heart failure. This is most usually caused by large left-to-right shunts (VSD, atrioventricular septal defect [AVSD], PDA) or myocardial failure (congenital cardiomyopathy or viral myocarditis). In this baby the blood pressure and clinical signs suggest that there is a coarctation. This prevents left ventricular emptying and so causes pulmonary oedema.

4. **J – Ventricular septal defect**
    VSDs give rise to left-to-right shunts. If big enough, the pulmonary overcirculation overwhelms the left ventricle and pulmonary oedema results. This makes the child tachypnoeic, increasing the work of breathing, and impedes feeding. The extra blood in the right ventricle increases the venous pressure and hepatomegaly, ascites and oedema will develop. The poor feeding and increased energy expenditure prevent weight gain. The bigger the VSD, the softer the murmur, because there will be less turbulence.

5.   C – Atrial septal defect
Fixed splitting is caused when left and right sides are connected by a septal defect. If there is a VSD, it cannot be heard behind the loud murmur. An atrial septal defect (ASD) allows blood to pass at low pressures from left to right and so does not give rise to a murmur directly. Instead, the increased blood flow in the right heart produces a flow murmur at the pulmonary valve.

13. INTERPRETATION OF PAEDIATRIC BLOOD GAS RESULTS

The list covers most of the major causes of acid–base disturbance in children. With knowledge of this and of the likely diseases at each age, this sort of question should be easy!

1.   D – Cyanotic congential heart disease
Here the child has a low PaO_2 despite being on 100% oxygen. There is no suggestion of respiratory distress, and the normal lactate level indicates that tissues are being well perfused. Cyanotic congential heart disease typically presents this way as there is reduced blood flow to the lungs, with venous blood entering the systemic circulation at a right-to-left shunt. The carbon dioxide levels are normal because it is much more diffusible than oxygen and so less pulmonary blood flow is needed to eliminate it.

2.   I – Pyloric stenosis
Vomiting boys aged 6–10 weeks are most likely to have pyloric stenosis in exams, although, in reality, gastro-oesophaeal reflux and a host of other causes are possible too. This baby has a metabolic alkalosis, with the beginnings of some respiratory compensation (the $PaCO_2$ is high-normal). This is because he has vomited acid. The tachycardia suggests cardiovascular compensation for hypovolaemia. It would be expected that the potassium would be low and the urine acidic. This is because potassium and hydrogen ions are lost in the urine in exchange for sodium ions in order to maintain the circulating volume.

3.   C – Bronchiolitis
This infant has an uncompensated respiratory acidosis, as well as tachypnoea and obvious respiratory problems. Carbon dioxide retention is most likely to be due to bronchiolitis in babies aged under 6 months and due to asthma in babies aged over 1 year. Here, small-airway obstruction prevents expiration more than inspiration, leading to hyperexpansion. CNS depressants such as barbiturates will also give rise to a respiratory acidosis, but there will be no respiratory signs.

4.   G – Inborn error of metabolism
Inborn errors of metabolism can present at any time during childhood, but most present in infancy. Severe forms present in the days after birth, when the placenta can no longer take away accumulated metabolic products. Presentations at this age will involve one or more of: acidosis, hypoglycaemia, hyperlactataemia or organic acids in the urine. Defects are commonly in amino acid-processing pathways, in the urea cycle or in mitochondrial function.

5. **A – Asthma**

This blood gas profile is near-normal, except for a low $PaCO_2$. This could be psychological, but the respiratory distress suggests pulmonary pathology. Even without looking at the gases, this is going to be asthma because this is the only respiratory problem affecting children at this age in the list.

14. DIAGNOSIS OF LOWER LIMB DISORDERS

Abnormal leg function is the end result of a number of musculoskeletal and neurological disorders. A comprehensive history and examination will identify most causes.

1. **I – Septic arthritis**

Children with pain in a joint or the limb will not want to move it, whatever the cause. If it is held rigidly, septic arthritis is most likely, although osteomyelitis and a fracture are also possible. The posture of flexion and external rotation at the hip is typical of a problem in the hip joint itself.

2. **J – Slipped femoral epiphysis**

If there is a discrepancy between true and apparent leg lengths, this is due to an asymmetric problem between the femoral shaft and the pelvis – congenital dislocation of the hip, slipped femoral epiphysis and fracture of the neck of femur are most likely. Active, and especially overweight adolescents put strain on the cartilage of the neck of the femur and make this group particularly prone to slipped femoral epiphysis. A fracture of the neck of the femur is unusual in children.

3. **A – Congenital dislocation of the hip**

At 3 years, such a discrepancy between true and apparent leg lengths is more likely to be due to congenital dislocation of the hip. Such hips are difficult to abduct, and there can be asymmetric skin creases in the thighs. Congenital dislocation of the hip should be picked up at the neonatal examination and at the 6-week check, using the Barlow and Ortolani tests.

4. **E – Osteomyelitis of the femur**

Following the reasoning in question 1, this child is likely to have osteomyelitis. It could also be a fracture of the shaft of the femur due to non-accidental injury, and this would be excluded with a radiograph. Osteomyelitis often cannot be seen in initial radiographs, becoming more obvious when the area becomes sclerotic. A radioisotope bone scan can be helpful.

5. **C – Duchenne's muscular dystrophy**

Hypertrophy of the calves is pathognomonic of Duchenne's muscular dystrophy, where there is damage to the muscle leading to swelling and fibrosis of the muscle. Boys with this X-linked recessive condition often are slow to learn to walk, then become more and more clumsy with time, eventually becoming wheelchair-bound. They typically die as a result of respiratory failure in their teens.

15. CAUSES OF ABNORMAL BREATH SOUNDS

Some senior physicians complain that clinical skills are being replaced by chest radiographs. There is some truth in this, and one should appreciate the limitations of auscultation – it only listens to the 5 cm or so under the stethescope, so in healthy lungs many areas are not heard at all; in small infants, the entire lung on one side can be heard without moving the stethescope at all! Chest radiographs supply additional and complementary information.

1. **B – Bronchiolitis**
Bilateral signs almost rule out pneumothorax (bilateral pneumothoraces are very unlikely), collapse and pneumonia, although viral pneumonia is frequently widespread. Bilateral signs are more often caused by asthma, bronchiolitis or pulmonary oedema. Expiratory problems in childhood are most often caused by asthma (over 1 year), bronchiolitis (under 6 months) or viral chest infections. Based on the findings and his age, this is likely to be bronchiolitis.

2. **I – Right pneumothorax**
This child has a tension pneumothorax and needs urgent drainage. They are more common in asthmatics and in tall and thin adolescents and can occur with severe pneumonia. A huge effusion might produce similar signs. Collapse of the left lung could deviate the trachea to the left, but breath sounds would also be reduced there.

3. **H – Pulmonary oedema**
Fine late-inspiratory crepitations result from the alveoli popping open at the part of the respiratory cycle with the greatest negative intrathoracic pressure. Respiratory distress syndrome, alveolitis and some pneumonias can cause this, but pulmonary oedema (from any cause) is most likely beyond the first few days of life.

4. **G – Left-sided pneumonia**
Pneumonia can manifest in a number of different signs. Consolidation assists conduction of sound from the bronchi to the surface, which can be heard as bronchial breathing or the sound of mucus moving along the airway.

5. **C – Inhaled foreign body in left main bronchus**
The signs are consistent with collapse of the left lung. Collapse can be due to mucus plugging, common in bronchiolitis and asthma, but can also be due to an inhaled foreign body. Depending on the item and where it lodges, foreign bodyies can produce a number of different signs and symptoms. Blockage at the larynx or carina can obstruct the airway completely, resulting in death. In the main-stem bronchi, air can sometimes pass into the lung, but exhalation is prevented, leading to unilateral hyperexpansion. Alternatively, the airway can become completely occluded, so that the lung beyond becomes de-gassed, collapsed or infected.

ANSWERS TO CHAPTER – RADIOLOGY

1. MUSCULOSKELETAL RADIOGRAPHS I – RADIOLOGICAL DIAGNOSIS

1. **1–3 H – Lytic lesin in the right femur**

    This radiograph shows a large lytic lesion in the proximal right femur, with further lesions within the pelvis. Lytic bone lesions are commonly associated with multiple myeloma and with lung, breast, thyroid and renal carcinoma. Prostate carcinoma can cause both lytic and sclerotic lesions, as can breast cancer.

2. **1–3 C – Pyrophosphate arthropathy**

    This radiograph shows intra-articular calcification of the left knee joint or 'chondrocalcinosis'. Causes include pyrophosphate arthropathy, primary hyperparathyroidism, haemochromatosis, hypophosphataemia and calcification of intra-articular structures following trauma.

3. **1–3 B – Paget's disease of bone**

    This radiograph shows severe Paget's bone disease of the skull, with gross and abnormal cortical thickening. This skull radiograph demonstrates 'platybasia', gross remodelling of the base of the skull, which in turn can cause compression of the lower brainstem and high cervical cord.

4. **1–3 D – Bamboo spine**

    This radiograph shows the characteristic 'bamboo spine' associated with ankylosing spondylitis. This appearance is caused by fusion of the vertebrae by syndesmophytes, which are caused by inflammation and ossification of the outer fibres of the annulus fibrosus.

5. **1–3 J – C1/C2 subluxation**

    This radiograph of the cervical spine shows atlanto-axial subluxation secondary to rheumatoid arthritis. This is potentially a surgical emergency and patients require urgent immobilisation and stabilisation of their cervical spine.

6. **1–3 G – Sclerotic lesion of L5**

    This radiograph of the lumbar spine shows a sclerotic lesion of L5. Causes include sclerotic metastasis from prostate or breast malignancy, chronic osteomyelitis, primary bone tumours and bone infarction.

2. MUSCULOSKELETAL RADIOGRAPHS II – CLINICAL DIAGNOSIS

1. **1–3 D – Bamboo spine**
   Ankylosing spondylitis is an idiopathic inflammatory disorder that is strongly associated with HLA-B27. It mainly affects the axial skeleton, particularly the sacroiliac and spinal facet joints. It also affects the ligaments and other paravertebral soft tissues. Radiologically, it produces the classic 'bamboo spine' (shown here) as a result of syndesmophyte formation.

2. **1–3 F – Gout**
   This radiograph shows tophaceous gout. Note the relative sparing of the proximal interphalangeal joints, with an asymmetrical degenerative arthropathy of the distal interphalangeal joints.

3. **1–3 G and H – Sclerotic lesion of L5 and a lytic lesion of the right femur**
   Radiograph **1–3 G** shows a solitary sclerotic lesion of L5; radiograph **1–3 H** shows multiple lytic lesions within the pelvis and right femur.

4. **1–3 B – Paget's disease of bone**
   This radiograph shows gross Paget's bone disease of the skull. Other bones commonly affected include the pelvis, femur, humerus, clavicles and vertebrae.

5. **1–3 E – Osteoarthritis**
   This radiograph shows an asymmetrical arthritis focused mainly around the distal interphalangeal joints, but also affecting both carpometacarpal joints. The proximal interphalangeal joints are spared. There is evidence of periarticualr sclerosis and loss of joint space in the right middle metacarpophalangeal joint, which is characteristic of osteoarthritis.

6. **1–3 C – Pyrophosphate arthropathy**
   This radiograph shows intra-articular calcification (chondrocalcinosis) of the left knee, commonly associated with pyrophosphate arthropathy. Pyrophosphate arthropathy or 'pseudogout' is more common in the elderly and it is important to differentiate it from gout because it does not respond to the gout prophylaxis (allopurinol). Aspiration of the joint and examination of the crystals under polarised light will demonstrate weakly positive birefringent crystals in pyrophosphate arthropathy and negatively birefringent crystals in gout.

3. MUSCULOSKELETAL RADIOGRAPHS III – CLINICAL SCENARIOS

1. **1–3 J – C1/C2 subluxation**
   This patient with rheuamtoid arthritis has developed a sinister complication, that of atlanto-axial subluxation. This is a neurosurgical emergency and the patient requires immediate immobilisation and stabilisation of the cervical spine. Neurosurgical decompression and stabilisation should be considered.

2. **1–3 C – Pyrophosphate arthropathy**

A monoarthirits in a man of this age is often mistaken for gout rather than the more common pyrophosphate arthropathy or 'pseudogout'. It is important to try and distinguish between the two because gout requires lifelong prophylaxis but pyrophosphate arthropathy does not. The single most effective differentiating test is examination of any affected joint's aspirate under polarised light. Gout produces negatively birefringent crystals while pyrophosphate arthropathy produces weakly positively birefringent crystals.

3. **1–3 B – Paget's disease of bone**

Paget's bone disease often presents with pain and immobility in the elderly. The characteristic gross elevation of the alkaline phosphatase must first be differentiated from that of hepatic alkaline phosphatase, excluded by normal liver function tests and in particular by a normal γGT. You should also exclude other bony causes, including fractures, metastases and osteomalacia, by checking the serum calcium and phosphate and by radiological investigation, including plain radiographs of painful areas and a bone scan if required.

4. **1–3 G (and 1–3 H) – Sclerotic lesion of L5 (and lytic lesion in the right femur)**

This gentleman has clinical features and investigations suggestive of metastatic prostate cancer. Radiograph **1–3 G** shows significant sclerotic change within L5, consistent with a metastatic deposit. It could be argued that radiograph **1–3 H**, which demonstrates multiple lytic lesions, could also be representative of his disease (although not really of his presenting symptoms; prostatic secondaries are also more commonly sclerotic).

5. **1–3 D – Bamboo spine**

This patient with long-standing ankylosing spondylitis now presents with the radiographic features of a 'bamboo spine'. Treatment remains symptomatic, with analgesia and physiotherapy. Note the family history of HLA-B27-associated disorders (inflammatory bowel disease and psoriasis).

4. GASTROENTEROLOGICAL RADIOLOGY I – CLINICAL DIAGNOSIS

1. **4–6 D – Achalasia**

This barium swallow shows the chactertic features of achalasia, an idiopathic disorder of the lower oesophagus that leads to an atonic lower segment. As it progresses this leads to pooling of food within the lower oesophagus which is commonly regurgitated unchanged. If left untreated, the condition is a risk for the development of malignancy in the lower oesophagus.

2. **4–6 H – Hiatus hernia**

This chest radiograph shows a large incarcerated hiatus hernia with a stomach bubble sitting behind the heart and leading to the apparent double heart border on the left.

3. **4–6 A, 4–6 E and 4–6 I – Linitis plastica, malignant ulcer and carcinoma of the colon**

These three radiological investigations show three very different malignant conditions. The barium meal in radiograph **4–6 A** shows the classic appearance of a 'leather bottle' stomach due to diffuse malignant invasion by a carcinoma of the stomach. This appearance is known as 'linitis plastica'. The barium meal in radiograph **4–6 E** demonstrates a large irregular ulcer on the lesser curvature of the stomach, representing a malignant ulcerative lesion of the stomach wall. Benign lesions usually appear as smooth-walled lesions. The barium enema of radiograph **4–6 I** demonstrates an 'apple core' lesion consistent with a malignancy in the transverse colon.

4. **4–6 F – Small-bowel obstruction**
    Radiograph **4–6 F** shows multiple fluid levels, a dilated stomach and small-bowel loops consistent with small-bowel obstruction. Common causes include postoperative adhesions, incarcerated inguinal and femoral hernias, Crohn's disease and malignancy.

5. **4–6 C – Lead piping**
    This double-contrast barium enema demonstrates loss of the haustral pattern ('lead piping') and pseudopolyposis affecting the transverse and descending colon. These changes are characteristic of ulcerative colitis.

6. **4–6 G – Diverticular disease**
    This barium enema demonstrates gross diverticulosis affecting most of the colon. Note that the patient was lying in the right-lateral position when this study was taken, as evidenced by the fluid levels on the left of the image.

5. GASTROENTEROLOGICAL RADIOLOGY II – CLINICAL SCENARIOS

1. **4–6 B – Pneumoperitoneum**
    This woman presents 24 hours after a routine laparoscopic procedure and has no signs to suggest that she is unwell or is suffering from any major complication. The finding of pneumoperitoneum is an expected one 24–48 hours after a laparoscopy. She should be reassured, given simple analgesia as required and sent home.

2. **4–6 I – Carcinoma of the colon**
    This man's history is suggestive of a colonic carcinoma, demonstrated by the barium enema in radiograph **4–6 I**. He has a microcytic anaemia and his deranged LFTs are suggestive of hepatic metastases. A CT scan of the abdomen should be arranged and further surgical and oncological management should be guided by the patient and by further radiological findings.

3. **4–6 G – Diverticular disease**
    This is a sinister history suggestive of colonic carcinoma, which needs to be excluded. Patients who do not want a colonoscopy (the investigation of choice) or a contrast-enhanced CT scan of the abdomen might agree to a barium study. This still requires the patient to take 24–36 hours of bowel preparation, be able to retain the enema, and be moved around the radiology couch in order to get adequate views. The three procedures need careful explanation before they are dismissed out of hand by anxious patients.

4. **4–6 F – Small-bowel obstruction**

This man has developed small-bowel obstruction, probably secondary to adhesions (in view of the multiple abdominal procedures). He requires adequate intravenous analgesia and an antiemetic, should be kept nil by mouth, should be 'dripped and sucked' (ie intravenous fluids, nasogastric tube insertion and aspiration of stomach contents) and started on intravenous antibiotics, and needs urgent surgical review. A CT scan of the abdomen might be useful for differentiating the possible underlying causes and will direct the future management.

5. **4–6 D – Achalasia**

This patient has developed symptoms of lower oesophageal dysphagia that are consistent with achalasia. The management should include barium swallow and/or upper gastrointestinal endoscopy to confirm the diagnosis. Once this has been achieved, symptomatic relief might be achieved with oral calcium-channel blockers or nitrates, and injection of botulinum toxin into the lower oesophageal sphincter. More radical treatments include balloon dilation of the sphincter or surgery. In patients well enough to undergo surgery, a laparoscopic Heller's procedure (myotomy) with partial fundoplication is a definitive procedure.

6. GASTROENTEROLOGICAL RADIOLOGY III – RADIOLOGICAL DIAGNOSIS

1. **4–6 I – Carcinoma of the colon**

This barium enema study demonstrates a severe malignant stricture of the transverse colon, commonly described as an 'apple core' lesion.

2. **4–6 C – Lead piping**

This is a double-contrast barium enema, which is used to demonstrate mucosal lesions. After a regular barium enema is administered, air is then introduced into the large bowel via the anus, so inflating the bowel and producing the 'double-contrast' effect. The mid- to distal transverse colon and descending colon in this study have lost their haustral pattern as a result of severe inflammatory bowel disease, producing the so-called 'lead piping' effect. The abnormal mucosa is also clearly seen.

3. **4–6 A – Linitis plastica**

This barium meal shows a grossly shrunken and abnormal stomach outline, linitis plastica, which is caused by diffuse invasion of the stomach by a malignancy. This in turn produces the so-called 'leather bottle' stomach seen on radiographs.

4. **4–6 D – Achalasia**

This barium swallow demonstrates proximal dilatation with severe tapering in the distal oesophagus, consistent with a 'bird's beak' deformity. This is produced by the atonic segment within the distal oesophagus, and is typical of achalasia. This appearance can also be seen in Chagas' disease, American trypanosomiasis.

5. **4–6 F and 4–6 J – Small-bowel obstruction and large-bowel obstruction**

Radiograph **4–6 F** is an erect abdominal radiograph which clearly demonstrates several fluid levels and pathologically dilated loops of small bowel. These are differentiated from the grossly dilated loops of large bowel seen in radiograph **4–6 J** by their plicae circulares and by the haustration of the loops in **4–6 J**.

6. **4–6 B – Pneumoperitoneum**
This erect abdominal radiograph shows gas under the right hemidiaphragm. This appearance, a pneumoperitoneum, can be caused by perforation of a hollow viscus, commonly associated with peritonitis. Iatrogenically, it might be produced through recent laparotomy or laparoscopy, peritoneal dialysis or paracentesis. In women, sexual intercourse, gynaecological examination and squatting exercises including ski-ing and water ski-ing can produce similar signs with no ill effects.

ANSWERS TO CHAPTER – SURGERY AND PATHOLOGY

1. INVESTIGATION OF ABDOMINAL PAIN

1.   F – General abdominal ultrasound
The clinical findings suggest gallstone disease. A general abdominal ultrasound includes the liver and biliary tree and is the investigation of choice in this scenario.

2.   C – CT scan
The clinical findings, taken with this man's associated risk factors, strongly suggest a diagnosis of dissecting abdominal aneurysm. The first step in investigation is a contrast CT scan to establish the diagnosis and the extent of the problem and thus plan surgical or endoprosthetic management.

3.   A – Chest and abdominal radiographs
The diagnosis that has to to be excluded first is that of perforated duodenal ulcer. An erect chest radiograph will demonstrate free gas in over 50% of patients with this diagnosis.

4.   A – Chest and abdominal radiographs
In this case a plain abdominal film can be used to make a diagnosis of large-bowel obstruction. Once this has been done in this case, a CT scan with rectal contrast or a gastrografin enema would then confirm the diagnosis and facilitate subsequent management (surgery or stenting).

5.   D – Diagnostic laparoscopy
This young woman's symptoms could be caused by appendicitis or could be related to a recurrence of her ovarian cystic pathology. Ovarian cysts can tort and infarct, or can rupture, leading to severe abdominal pain and low-grade fever, which can closely mimic the signs and symptoms of appendicitis. In the face of such uncertainty, a diagnostic laparoscopy is appropriate so that either condition can be managed, and the increased use of this investigation has led to a reduction in the rate of negative appendicectomy. A pelvic ultrasound scan would be more appropriate when you suspect that a patient has an acute condition that does not require surgery.

2. FAECAL INCONTINENCE

Put simply, faecal incontinence can be thought of as a disturbance either to the passage or to the passenger. The 'passage' consists of the rectum (storage) and the anal canal, which is composed of two rings of muscle (the internal and external anal sphincters) whose function can be disturbed by direct injury or by neuropathy of the pudenal nerve (a mixed nerve that provides motor function to the external anal sphincter). The 'passenger' (ie faeces), if loose, can result in incontinence, even in the presence of a normally functioning anorectal sphincteric complex.

1. **G – Sphincter disruption**
Obstetric trauma frequently results in a transient degree of faecal incontinence in the immediate post-partum period in up to a third of women, but generally subsequently improves. This is related to traction of the sphincteric complex and the pudendal nerve. An alarming proportion of women sustain occult sphincteric damage and the evidence suggests that many third-degree tears (extending from perineum to involve the anal sphincter complex) are inadequately repaired.

2. **B – Colorectal carcinoma**
In this case the 'passenger' is responsible for causing faecal incontinence. The scenario highlights the importance of excluding all organic pathology in a patient with new symptoms and change in bowel habit.

3. **F – Pudendal neuropathy**
Multiple, traumatic vaginal deliveries will result in a stretch injury to the pudendal nerve. This results in a weakness in the external anal sphincter, causing attenuated squeeze pressure. Patients subsequently complain of an inability to defer defaecation (urgency) with incontinence.

4. **D – Faecal impaction**
Incontinence is extremely common in people living in nursing homes. In many patients this is as a result of impaction of a large bolus of hard faeces in the rectum, which leads to distortion of the anal canal and leakage of liquid faeces past the bolus. Treatment is directed at avoiding constipation.

5. **A – Acute gastroenteritis**
The history is typical of this condition. The problem here is the passenger. Incontinence is possible with severe diarrhoea in all but those with the most 'titanic' sphincter.

3. GROIN LUMPS

1. **F – Inguinal hernia**
This requires little explanation. The history, reducibility and position point to this diagnosis.

2. **G – Inguinal lymphadenopathy**
The findings indicate this diagnosis. In this case, the likely diagnosis is of a sexually transmitted disease, for example lymphogranuloma venereum infection, and appropriate investigations should be performed. Painless, more enlarged nodes should prompt a search for other causes. Remember that the lower limb, anus and external genitalia all drain to the groin.

3. **H – Psoas abscess**
Although this mass could be attributed to lymphadenopathy, the fluctuant nature and the presence of ipsilateral hip pain point to a diagnosis of psoas abscess. Psoas abscesses develop either from infection of unknown origin or as a consequence of infection spreading from an adjacent organ (usually bowel or urinary tract). Treatment is now usually (initially at least) by percutaneous drainage under ultrasound or CT guidance, with antibiotic treatment of the infecting organism (in this case the abscess has probably originated from a tuberculous spine).

4. **D – Femoral hernia**
    This woman has signs of small-bowel obstruction secondary to a strangulated femoral hernia. A small complicated hernia in the groin crease in an elderly person with no prior history of a reducible lump is much more likely to be a femoral hernia than an inguinal hernia (although inguinal hernias are approximately ten times more common, in general).

5. **B – False aneurysm**
    The nature of this man's investigation points to the diagnosis of a false aneurysm. Failure to compress the site of arterial cannulation (a traumatic breach in the vessel wall) leads to extravasation of arterial blood. A haematoma then forms in the soft tissues around the artery, which produces a transmissible pulse. A true aneurysm is one that involves all of the layers of the arterial wall and is often expansile.

4. POSTOPERATIVE HYPOXIA

1. **K – Upper airway obstruction**
    This is one of the specific complications of thyroid surgery (the others being dysphonia, hypocalcaemia and hypothyroidism). It can be caused by haematoma formation under the strap muscles of the neck with compression of the airway, bilateral recurrent laryngeal neuropraxia or tracheomalacia. Emergency intervention is required.

2. **B – Basal atelectasis**
    Postoperative atelectasis is commonly observed in the early post-operative period, especially after prolonged surgery with the patient in the supine position; diaphragmatic dysfunction and reduced surfactant are consequences of general anaesthesia. In addition, inadequate analgesia leads to reduced respiratory excursion and coughing. The resultant hypoventilation of the lung bases leads to localised small-airway collapse and is usually accompanied by a low-grade pyrexia.

3. **J – Pulmonary oedema**
    This is due to increased hydrostatic pressure (eg volume overload – as in this scenario, and left ventricular failure). Fluid accumulates around the lung parenchyma, especially in the dependant basal regions of the lower lobes, causing alveolar collapse. It is not uncommon in postoperative patients, in whome it can be due to injudicious intravenous fluid administration. A peri-operative cardiac event should be excluded however.

4. **F – Pleural effusion**
    Fluid in the pleural space can be: (1) a transudate (<30 g/l of protein), secondary to either increased hydrostatic pressure (eg from volume overload or left ventricular failure) or decreased oncotic pressure (eg from hypoalbunaemia, as in this scenario); or (2) an exudate (>30 g/l protein), secondary to capillary hyperpermeability (resulting from malnutrition, carcinoma or Gram-negative sepsis). Fluid fills the basal aspect of the pleural space, inhibiting lung expansion.

5. **A – Adult respiratory distress syndrome**
    Adult respiratory distress syndrome, or non-cardiogenic pulmonary oedema, is often an early manifestation of the systemic inflammatory response syndrome (SIRS) and,

later, of the multiorgan dysfunction syndrome (MODS). It is the manifestation of progressive combined ventilatory, perfusion and diffusional pathology. Pulmonary capillary leakage results in impaired oxygen diffusion and reduced lung compliance, In addition, leakage into the alveoli leads to the hyalination and fibrosis that are responsible for the characteristic radiological appearance of bilateral pulmonary infiltrates.

5. POSTOPERATIVE OLIGURIA

1. D –Haemorrhagic shock
Postoperative bleeding can occur after aortic aneurysm surgery. The clinical signs in this case give the diagnosis. Treatment can be re-operative or by intensive monitoring and support.

2. B – Cardiogenic shock
This gentleman is diabetic and an arteriopath, as indicated by his admission for vascular bypass surgery. His poor urine output, compromised blood pressure (with no clear evidence of overt or covert haemorrhage) and the vague history of 'indigestion'-type pain that has not settled with antacids suggest a coronary cause for his hypotension and oliguria. This is confirmed by a failure of fluid bolus replacement to sustain a rise in blood pressure. This man needs a thorough cardiovascular assessment (including ECG, chest radiograph, general bloods, cardiac enzymes and, probably, central venous pressure measurement). If he has had a myocardial infarct, clearly he will be unable to undergo thrombolysis as this is contraindicated by the recent vascular surgery. Instead, treatment (preferably on the Coronary Care Unit) should be supportive (oxygen, analgesia) and inotropes should be started if his hypotension fails to improve.

3. E – Increased ADH secretion
This forms part of the normal physiological response to trauma (in this case, surgery). In the simplest analysis, water is retained by the kidney as a protective response. The situation resolves spontaneously by approximately 48 hours after the trauma. Management is the exclusion of other causes of oliguria.

4. I – Urinary retention
Never forget this as a cause of oliguria – remember that the causes are pre-renal, renal and post-renal, the latter being the case here, where the urinary catheter has become blocked. This is suggested by the pattern of decline in urine output and the presence of normal and stable vital signs in the presence of anuria.

6. ADVANCES RELATED TO SURGERY

1. I – James Paget (1814–1889)
James Paget was a St Bartholomew's Hospital surgeon who published over 20 articles on various aspects of pathology and surgery. He was one of the first surgeons to correlate patients' symptoms with the clinical examination and developed many of the ideas of clinical surgery. Amongst his achievements, he described Paget's disease of the nipple (caused by underlying cancer) and osteitis deformans (Paget's disease of bone).

2. **J – John Snow (1813–1858)**

    John Snow was a British physician and surgeon and a leader in the adoption of anaesthesia and medical hygiene. He is often also considered to be the father of epidemiology because of his work in tracing the source of a cholera outbreak in London. In 1853 he administered chloroform anaesthesia to Queen Victoria, bringing about its widespread acceptance (its first use was attributed to James Simpson).

3. **G – Karl Landsteiner (1868–1943)**

    An Austrian pathologist who made numerous contributions to pathological anatomy, histology and immunology. His name is best known in association with his discovery in 1901 of (and outstanding work on) blood groups, the basis for blood transfusion, for which he was awarded the Nobel Prize for Physiology or Medicine in 1930.

4. **A – Christian Theodor Billroth (1829–1894)**

    A German-Austrian surgeon who is considered the founder of modern abdominal surgery. Billroth introduced epoch-making treatments which formed the pattern for surgical operations of the stomach, biliary tract, and female genitalia for several decades. As professor of the Vienna School of Surgery and because of his own work and that of his many eminent pupils, he probably was the single most influential figure in the development of modern surgical knowledge.

5. **D – William Halstead (1852–1922)**

    An American surgeon who published a technique of inguinal hernia repair and described the radical mastectomy for breast cancer, which his name is associated with. Halstead was a great surgical educator who, influenced by his early years in Germany (with Billroth), introduced a formal training programme for junior surgeons. He was the founder of the surgical training programme at the Johns Hopkins University that was subsequently used as the model for many other teaching systems.

7.   ENTERAL AND PARENTERAL NUTRITION

1. **C – Feeding jejunostomy**

    Most surgeons choose to form a feeding jejunostomy at surgery. Feeding is instigated until a gastrografin swallow demonstrates an intact anastomosis and oral nutrition can be restarted.

2. **F – Low-volume, low-electrolyte diet**

    This patient requires a low-volume, low-electrolyte feed (ie low sodium and low potassium). Patients with chronic renal failure, which is controlled in this patient by continuous ambulatory peritoneal dialysis, are unable to eliminate high-volume feeds adequately and the resulting fluid overload can precipitate peripheral oedema and cardiac failure.

3. **K – Percutaneous endoscopic gastrostomy (PEG) feeding**

    Patients who requireg tube feeding for periods of more than a month should have a more permanent form of feeding tube inserted. This is to prevent the inevitable problems that can occur with chronic use of a nasoenteric tube (patient discomfort, sinusitis and epistaxis).

4. **E – Intravenous nutrition**
    The average length of the adult human small intestine has been found to be approximately 600 cm from studies performed on cadavers. Any disease, traumatic injury, vascular accident, or other pathological process that leaves less than 200 cm of viable small bowel places the patient at risk of developing short-bowel syndrome; with less than 100 cm, problems are inevitable, especially if there is no colonic absorption of water (as in this case). Some form of intravenous nutrition (usually total parenteral nutrition) is required, at least for an initial period. With time, it is often possible to re-institute some form of enteral nutrition in combination the intravenous route.

5. **I – Nasojejunal feeding**
    Recent studies have supported the use of early enteral nutrition in pancreatitis, including severe cases. The basic premise is that feeding helps to maintain the epithelial barrier, so reducing bacterial translocation and subsequent SIRS or MODS. While some have tried nasogastric feeding, most of these patients have experienced nausea and vomiting with this type of feeding.

8. TYPES OF SHOCK

1. **E – Neurogenic shock**
    This results from impairment of descending sympathetic pathways in the spinal cord, with loss of vasomotor tone and hence vasodilatation of splanchnic/lower-extremity blood vessels. It should not be confused with spinal shock, which refers to the flaccidity and loss of reflexes seen acutely after spinal injury.

2. **B – Cardiogenic**
    This patient has Beck's classic triad of tachycardia, muffled heart sounds and engorged neck veins, with hypotension resistant to fluid therapy suggesting cardiac tamponade. Cardiac tamponade, a well-recognised cause of cardiogenic shock, results in impairment of cardiac function and failure of the heart to maintain the circulation as a result of 'pump failure'. It has a 90% mortality, prompt pericardiocentesis providing the only relief.

3. **C – Haemorrhagic**
    From the presentation, this patient probably has a leaking abdominal aortic aneurysm. The findings indicate a 30–40% blood volume loss (approximately 2000 ml in a 70-kg adult), defined as a class III haemorrhage.

4. **G – Septic**
    Circulating endotoxins, commonly from Gram-negative organisms, cause vasodilatation – leading to a widened pulse pressure and warm peripheries – and impair energy utilisation at a cellular level. Tissue hypoxia can occur, even with normal or high oxygen delivery rates, because of the increased tissue oxygen demands and direct impairment of cellular oxygen uptake. In addition, the endotoxin causes capillary wall hyperpermeability, worsened by the stimulation of proteolytic enzymes, leading to poorly controlled fluid transfer from the intravascular space to the interstitial space, effectively resulting in hypovolaemia. The situation is aggravated by the negatively inotropic effect of bacterial endotoxin on the myocardium.

5. **C – Haemorrhagic**
This is a bit of a trick question for all those who thought the answer would be anaphylactic shock. In a polytrauma patient, the cause of shock is always hypovolaemic until proved otherwise. When injuries to the chest, pelvis and lower extremity are evident, it is very likely that there is internal haemorrhage in the abdomen and/or pelvis.

9. MANAGEMENT DECISIONS IN TRAUMA CARE

1. **D – Chest, pelvic and lateral cervical spine radiographs**
These are the first investigations performed as adjuncts to the primary survey and resuscitation. The lateral cervical spine radiograph is now sometimes omitted in favour of CT scanning.

2. **I – Focused assessment with sonography for trauma (FAST) scan**
This is a relatively recent addition to the tests that are available during trauma calls and which in some ways has replaced diagnostic peritoneal lavage (although there are still some instances where this is useful). The ultrasound probe is used in five areas in order to assess for abdominal (four areas) and pericardial (one area) fluid. It is a very rapid test that can be performed by trained non-radiological personnel. It gives no information beyond the detection of free fluid.

3. **E – CT scan**
In this situation, because the patient remains stable, you have the opportunity to gain further information about intra-abdominal injuries by performing a CT scan (often the chest and neck are also included to further exclude injuries). It should be emphasised that the patient must be stable and have an appropriate accompanying team, as well as adequate resuscitation facilities available in the imaging unit – the CT scanner is known as the 'doughnut of death' by some trauma surgeons for good reason. CT imaging is excellent for assessing the extent of organ damage, retroperitoneal injury and pelvic organ injury and so is also extremely useful for assisting decision-making regarding operative intervention. It has an accuracy of 92–98% but can miss small diaphragmatic and bowel injuries.

4. **G – Emergency laparotomy**
Whilst awaiting the CT scan, the patient has become unstable. Given that you know that there is free fluid in the abdomen (from the FAST scan), you should proceed immediately to surgery. Given the left flank bruising, the likely diagnosis is a splenic injury.

10. INVESTIGATION AND MANAGEMENT OF GASTROINTESTINAL DISEASE

1. **G – Double-contrast barium enema**
There are perhaps three options here, where the index of suspicion of significant pathology is low. At one extreme, it might be reasonable not to investigate at all or just to perform a plain abdominal radiograph (and treat accordingly). At the other extreme, you could order a colonoscopy, although this is not without risk of complications and

has availability/cost implications. A barium enema will exclude significant pathology with reasonable sensitivity and can diagnose diverticular disease.

2. **J – Oesophagogastroduodenoscopy (OGD) and adrenaline (epinephrine) injection**
    In such a situation it is recommended that haemostasis is attempted with injection of 1 : 10 000 adrenaline (epinephrine). Although evidence-based practice has shown heat-probe or bipolar diathermy and injection sclerotherapy all to be effective, adrenaline injection is often used in combination with these modalities, and available trials show that adrenaline alone is equally effective. Only if this fails or if there are other endoscopic or clinical indications should the patient undergo surgery (under-running of the ulcer).

3. **M – Proctosigmoidoscopy**
    This is the first investigation of choice and will reveal the cause (eg piles) in many cases. If no evident cause is found in the anorectum and fresh bleeding continues, flexible sigmoidoscopy would be the next step. In contrast, dark-red bleeding or melaena, or an associated change in bowel habit (to loose stools or diarrhoea) would favour the performance of a full colonoscopy.

4. **C – Bidirectional endoscopy**
    In this instance (a microcytic anaemia without an obvious cause), OGD followed by colonoscopy are indicated to try to find a cause for the anaemia. If these fail to locate a cause, a capsule (wireless) endoscopy could be indicated.

5. **A – Angiography**
    This woman has ongoing small-bowel/proximal colonic haemorrhage (melaena plus dark fresh blood). Although ultimately she might require a laparotomy/colectomy, the next, intermediate step is to perform an emergency mesenteric angiogram. This can localise bleeding in 58–86% of patients who have active bleeding (classified as a rate of 1–1.5 ml/minute). Red-cell scanning can detect slower bleeds but with little accuracy in terms of localisation. Angiography also allows immediate therapeutic intervention with embolisation using metal microcoils or gelfoams. If these attempts fail, an emergency laparotomy, with on-table endoscopy/enteroscopy, should be performed.

Self-assessment EMQ Papers

List of EMQ Test questions – 10 Exams of 12 Questions for each Volume

Ten practice examinations of 12 questions are listed below, drawing questions from across the syllabus: each is intended as a two-hour examination.

VOLUME 2

1. 1.2; 1.14, 1.22; 2.7; 2.17; 3.2; 3.14; 3.24; 4.10; 5.2; 5.12; 7.1
2. 1.3; 1.15; 1.24; 2.8; 2.18; 3.4; 3.15; 4.1; 4.11; 5.3; 5.13; 7.3
3. 1.4; 1.12; 1.25; 2.9; 2.19; 3.5; 3.16; 4.2; 4.12; 5.4; 5.14; 7.4
4. 1.5; 1.13; 1.26; 2.10; 2.20; 3.6; 3.17; 4.3; 4.13; 5.5; 5.15; 7.5
5. 1.6; 1.16; 1.27; 2.11; 2.21; 3.7; 3.18; 4.4; 4.14; 5.6; 6.1; 7.6
6. 1.7; 1.17; 1.28; 2.12; 2.22; 3.9; 3.19; 4.5; 4.15; 5.7; 6.4; 7.7
7. 1.8; 1.18; 2.3; 2.13; 2.23; 3.10; 3.20; 4.6; 4.16; 5.8; 6.5; 7.8
8. 1.9; 1.19; 2.4; 2.14; 2.24; 3.11; 3.21; 4.7; 4.17; 5.9; 6.2; 7.9
9. 1.10; 1.20; 2.5; 2.15; 2.25; 3.12; 3.22; 4.8; 4.18; 5.10; 6.3; 7.2
10. 1.11; 1.21; 2.6; 2.16; 3.1; 3.13; 3.23; 4.9; 5.1; 5.11; 6.6; 7.10

Index

All references are to chapter and theme number, e.g. 1.8 refers to Chapter 1, Theme 8